Rika Singh
Akanksha Singh

MATRIX METALLOPROTEINASES IN HEALTH AND DISEASE

Rika Singh
Akanksha Singh

MATRIX METALLOPROTEINASES IN HEALTH AND DISEASE

Regulators of Tissue Remodeling and Disease Progression

LAP LAMBERT Academic Publishing

Imprint

Any brand names and product names mentioned in this book are subject to trademark, brand or patent protection and are trademarks or registered trademarks of their respective holders. The use of brand names, product names, common names, trade names, product descriptions etc. even without a particular marking in this work is in no way to be construed to mean that such names may be regarded as unrestricted in respect of trademark and brand protection legislation and could thus be used by anyone.

Cover image: www.ingimage.com

Publisher:
LAP LAMBERT Academic Publishing
is a trademark of
Dodo Books Indian Ocean Ltd. and OmniScriptum S.R.L publishing group

120 High Road, East Finchley, London, N2 9ED, United Kingdom
Str. Armeneasca 28/1, office 1, Chisinau MD-2012, Republic of Moldova, Europe
Managing Directors: Ieva Konstantinova, Victoria Ursu
info@omniscriptum.com

Printed at: see last page
ISBN: 978-620-8-44226-2

INDEX

Introduction

Matrix metalloproteinases (MMPs) are metal binding proteins derived from mesenchymal cells, hematopoietic cells including monocytes and macrophages, and keratinocytes that degrade various proteins in the extracellular matrix.[1] MMPs are members of the metzincin protease superfamily of zinc and calcium dependent preteolytic enzymes.[2] The prototype of host- derived, connective tissue destructive matrix metalloproteinases, namely interstitial collagenase, was first reported in 1962, by James Gross and Charles Lapiere after their study on tadpole tail resorption during metamorphosis.[3] Metalloproteinases can synergistically digest all the macromolecules of tissue matrices, although they are not necessarily produced together.[4] These proteinases are involved in a variety of physiological events such as embryonic development, involving of the post-partum uterus, tissue remodelling, salivary gland morphogenesis and tooth eruption. In addition, they also play a role in pathological processes such as periodontal disease, arthritis, cancer, atherosclerosis, diabetes pulmonary emphysema and osteoporosis.[5]

Connective tissue remodelling is an integral part of normal growth and development. These endopeptidase are principle enzymes in degenerative processes, since the protein components of most matrix macromolecules are the predominant determinants of tissue structure and function.[1] An important feature of metalloproteinases is that they are secreted in latent forms. The latent form needs to be activated before it can exert its function. The pro-forms have a pro-peptide containing a conserved cystine in a region of homology. The activation of latent enzyme occurs through dissociation of cysteine that is bonded to the zinc of active site leading to exposure of active side.[6]

MMPs are anchored to cell surface thus restricting their activities to membrane proteins or proteins in the extracellular space.[1] MMPs regulate the functions of a variety of biologically active molecules like growth factors, serine protease inhibitors and pro- inflammatory molecules like cytokines, chemokines.[7] All major cells in the periodontal tissues are capable of synthesizing and releasing different MMPs when activated.[8] The production of MMPs is amplified in periodontal lesion by signals transmitted by various cells. This leads to accelerated breakdown of periodontal tissues. Birkedal- Hansen gave the evidence for the role of MMPs in tissue destruction in periodontal disease. It has been summarised as follows:

1) MMPs were expressed by cells isolated from normal and inflamed gingiva.

2) GCF samples from gingivitis and periodontitis patients have shown presence of MMP-8 and MMP-3.[9]

MMPs play a critical role in connective tissue turnover. Molecular pathways critical to regulation of MMP gene transcription, MMP synthesis and activation of latent MMP molecules led to the discovery of endogenous inhibitors of these molecules which came to be known as tissue inhibitors of matrix metalloproteinases (TIMPs).[10] TIMPs there are additional mechanisms that fine tune the activities of MMPs including mRNA stability, cell surface recruitment, enzyme compartmentalization, shedding, oligomerization, cellular uptake and autolysis. It is important for these mechanisms to operate in a coordinated manner so that MMP expression is well balanced. A study done on rabbit models with arthritis showed a decline in TIMP synthesis as compared to MMPs in synovial explants.[11] This study gave the first evidence that destruction of tissue in disease processes might be as result of imbalance between MMPs and TIMPs. Endogenous inhibitors of metalloproteinases bind in a high affinity, irreversible non- covalent manner to inhibit MMPs.[12] They bind to the active sites of MMPs. TIMPs are expressed by a number of periodontal cells and osteoblasts.[13]

Historical Background

In the year 1962, Jerome Gross and Chales Lapiere showed production of a collagenolytic factor in the skin, gut and gills of animal tadpole. These tissues underwent radical remodelling during metamorphosis. The collagenolytic factor worked at a neutral pH and physiologic temperature resulting in degradation of denatured collagen in living animal tissue culture.[14] Thus MMP was first identified in 1962 by this milestone study. In 1966, MMP-1 was purified from tadpole tail fin and back skin.[15] Before this study there was another study by Woessner in 1962, this study done on mammalian uterus showed that a protein enzyme could degrade collagen. The metabolic breakdown of collagen and non-collagen protein was studied in the rat uterus undergoing post partum involution.[16] MMP-2 which was initially denoted as 72-kDa type IV collagenase/ gelatinase A, was first isolated and described in the 1970s.[17] In 1988, Goldberg and colleagues sequenced MMP-2. This enzyme was referred to as type IV collagenase because it could digest type IV collagen in the basement membrane.[18] In 1990, Yasunori Okada et al did a study on human synovial tissue which was obtained at anthroplasty from patients with rheumatoid arthritis. They cultured fibroblasts with rabbit alveolar macrophage conditioned medium. They were isolated and purified MMP-2 in its inactive form, pro MMP2. They further studied the activation and enzymatic activities of MMP-2.[19]

The first description of proteinase activity of MMP-3 came during the 1970s.[17] A study done by Galloway WA in 1983 purified MMP-3, also known as 'proteoglycanase' from rabbit bone culture. The purification of MMP-3 enabled the analysis of its activity on individual connective tissue components and to assess its potential role in physiological remodelling and pathological destruction.[20]

Additional MMPs were identified over years and Ed Harris Jr and colleagues proposed the name matrix metalloproteinases in the late 1980.[21] Subsequently the International Union of Biochemistry and Molecular Biology designated the family with the name 'MMP' and assigned each enzyme a number. By 1991, MMP- 1,2,3,7,8,9 and 10 had been named and characterised. MMPs have been classified into five subgroups: collagenases, gelatinases, matrilysins, stromelysins and membrane type MMPs based on sequence homology and in vitro extracellular matrix substrate characteristics. An MMP should have following characteristics:[22]

1. Proteolysis of at least one extracellular matrix component.
2. Catalysed by zinc present at the active site.
3. To be activated by proteinases or organomercurials.
4. Should be inhibited by ethylene diaminetetraacetic acid 1, 10-phenanthroline and one of the TIMPs.
5. cDNA has sequence homology to MMP-1.[23]

Lovejoy and colleagues in 1994 gave the first crystal structure of human fibroblast collagenase catalytic domain.[24] The crystal structure was solved in the form of a collagenase- inhibitor complex at a resolution of 2.4 Å. Following this the 3D structure of catalytic domains were determined by x-ray crystallography by several groups.[25-27] Subsequently in 1995, crystal structure of pro-MMP-3 lacking the hemopexin domain was given by JW Becket and colleagues. They determined the three dimensional structure of C- truncated form of the pro enzyme and an inhibited complex of the catalytic domain by x-ray diffraction analysis.[28] In the same year, J Li et al studied the crystal structure of full length MMP-1 at 2.5 Å resolution. They found that the catalytic domain and haemopexin like of 17 amino acids. The catalytic domain contains three calcium binding sites and the haemopexin like domain contains four units of four stranded anti-parallel beta sheets. The beta sheet is stabilized by a cation, probably calcium. Since then structures of other MMPs have been determined using x-ray crystalline and by NMR spectroscopy.[29]

Classification

On the basis of structure and substrate specificity MMPs have been divided into six groups.

Collagenases:

They are enzymes that break the peptide bonds in collagen. The term was first used by Gross and Lapiere in 1962 when they demonstrated presence of enzyme that dissolved highly protease- resistant matrix constituting collagen fibrils. It marked the beginning of an existing period of discovery that led to the identification of a large number of distinct metalloproteinases.[3]

Collagenase - 1

- Also numerically classified as MMP-1
- Chromosomal location: 11q22-q23[30]
- Biological effect: Migration of keratinocytes, re-epithelialisation, cell migration, platelet aggregation, increase in the bioavailability of IGF-1, cell proliferation, pro- inflammatory effect, PARP1 activation, in cancer progression.[31,32]
- Group of substrates for enzymes: Collegen (I, II, III, VIII), casein, intactin, laminin, pro MMP- 1,2,9 [30]

Collagenase - 2

- Also numerically classified as MMP-8
- Chromosomal location: 11q22- q23 [30]
- Biological effect: Activation of osteoclasts, enhancement of collagen affinity in cancer progression, cleavage of α and β chemokines and regulation of their mobilization.[31,32]

- Group of substrates for enzymes: Collagen (I, III, V, VII, X), gelatin, fibronectin.[30]

Collagenase - 3

- Also numerically classified as MMP-13
- Chromosomal location: 11q 22.3[30]
- Biological effect: In cancer progression- induction of EMT, cell migration[31]

Gelatinases:

They are neutral MMPs requiring Ca2+ for activity and are involved in the proteolysis and disruption of basement membrane by degradation of type IV, type V and denatures collgens. There are 2 types of gelatinases:

1. 72 kDa gelatinase[30] - Gelatinase A
2. 92 kDa gelatinase[31] – Gelatinase B [33]

72 kDa gelatinase has been found complexed to TIMP-2,[34] whereas the 92 kDa gelatinase has been complexed to TIMP-1.[35]

Gelatinase - A

- Also numerically classified as MMP-2
- Chromosomal location: 16q13 [30]
- Biological effect: growth of axons, cell migration, differentiation of mesenchymal cell with inflammation phenotype, enhancement of collagen affinity, cell proliferation, migration of epithelial cells, increase in TGF- β, neuronal apoptosis leading to neurodegeneration [31,32] .

- Group of substrates for enzymes: Gelatin, collagen (IV, V,VII, X, XIV), elastin, fibrillin, osteonectin [30]

Gelatinase - B

- Also numerically classified as MMP-9
- Chromosomal location: 20q 11. 2q 13.1 [30]
- Biological activity: Collagen affinity enhancing, pro-inflammatory and anti- inflammatory activity, tumor cell resistance, IL-2 response reduction, incorporation of new units of functional osteoblasts.[31,32]
- Group of substrates for enzymes:Gelatin, collagen (IV, V, VII, X, XIV), elastin, osteonectin.[30]

Stromelysins:

They have a broad substrate specificity for components of ECM. Has an estimate molecular weight of 54kDa. Mesenchymal cells, such as chondrocytes and fibroblasts are commonly found to secrete stromelysin 1.[36] Transin, the rat homologue of human stromelysin, was originally discovered in fibroblasts transformed with the polyvirus.[37]

Stomelysin - 1

- Also numerically classified as MMP-3
- Chromosomal location: 11q23. [30]
- Biological activity: Migration of cells, epithelial cell apoptosis, epithelial mesenchymal conversion, angiostatin- like elements generation, release of bFGF, increase in bioavailability of IGF-1, cell proliferation, increase in bioavailability of TGF- β, increase in cell invasiveness, up regulation of angiogenesis.[31,32]

- Group of substrates for enzymes: Laminin, gelatin, fibronectin.[30]

Stromelysin - 2

- Also numerically classified as MMP-10
- Chromosomal location: 11q 22.3- q23.[30]
- Biological activity: In cancer progression, generation of tumstatin, endostatin, angiostain.[32]
- Group of substrates for enzymes: Collagen (III- V), gelatine, elastin, casein.[30]

Stromelysin- 3

- Also numerically classified as MMP-11
- Chromosomal location: 22q 11.2[30]
- Biological activity: Is expressed in tissues undergoing active remodelling associated with embryonic development, wound healing and tumor invasion. It may promote tumourogenicity[31,32].
- Group of substrates for enzymes: Fibronectin, laminin, aggregan, gelatine[30]

Matrilysin:

The name matrilysin denotes lysis of matrix . They are capable of digesting a large series of proteins of the extracellular matrix, demonstrating preference for Leu of Ile in the P1 position in the exposed regions between structural domains to produce multiple fragments. They also degrade matrix proteoglycans and glycoproteins.[36]

- Also numerically classified as MMP-7
- Chromosomal location: 11q 21- q 22[30]
- Biological activity: Adipocyte differenciation, collagen affinity enhancement, an increase in cell invasiveness, abnormal cell aggregation, activation of osteoclasts.

Cleaves a variety of secreted and cell surface proteins including growth factors and growth factor binding proteins, cell surface receptors, apoptosis factors, cell adhesion molecules, MMP-7 can release active forms of cellular signalling molecules such as TNF-α family members.[31,32]

- Group of substrates for enzymes: Collagen (IV- X), fibronectin, laminin, gelatine, aggregan, pro- MMP-9.[30]

Metalloelastase

- Also numerically classified as MMP-12
- Chromosomal location: 11q 22.2 q 22.3.[30]
- Biological activity: MMP-12, a protease involved in macrophage migration, could also have a crutial role in regulating the resolution of inflammation. MMP-12 degrades elastin and is highly expressed by macrophages and other stromal cells, also found in hypertonic chondrocytes and osteoclasts.[3]
- Group of substrates for enzymes: Elastin, gelatin, collagen (I, IV), fibronectin, laminin, vibronectin, proteoglycan.[30]

Matrilysin - 2

- Also numerically classified as MMP-26
- Chromosomal location: 11p 15.[30]
- Biological activity: Demonstrates proteolytic activity toward several substrates including type IV collagen, β casein, fibrinogen, fibronectin, gelatine. It also

activates pro- MMP-9. The broad proteolytic activity and distribution of MMP- 26 in different cell lines suggest that it may play a role in tissue remodelling events associated with angiogenesis and tumor progression.[31,32]

- Group of substrates for enzymes: Gelatin, collagen (IV), pro-MMP-9.[30]

Membrane type MMPs

MT- MMPs include four transmembrane MMPs, MMP-14,15,16,24 and two glycosal phophatidylinositol (GP1) anchored MMPs, MMP 17 and 25. They are activated intracellularly and the active enzymes expressed on the cell surface MT- MMPs have membrane-anchoring domains and display protease activity at the cell surface and therefore they are optimal pericellular proteolytic machines.[38] All MT-MMPs except MT4- MMP can activate pro MMP 2.[39]

MT- MMP - 1

- Also numerically classified as MMP-14
- Chromosomal location- 14q 11-q12.[30]
- Biological activity: Anti-inflammatory action, epithelial cell migration, collagenolytic activity, digesting type I, II, II collagens into characteristic ¾ and
  ¼ fragment. The activity of MT1- MMP on type I collagen is synergistically increased with coincubation with MMP-2.[31]
- Group of substrates for enzymes: Collagen (I, II, III), gelatine, fibronectin, laminin, aggrecan, tenascin.[30]

MT- MMP - 2

- Also numerically classified as MMP-15
- Chromosomal location: 15p 13- q12.[30]

- Biological activity: It is essential for pericellular matrix remodelling in late stages of development as well as in growth and tissue homeostasis in post natal life.[31,32]
- Group of substrates for enzymes:
- Fibronectin, laminin, aggrecan, perlecan.[30]

MT- MMP - 3

- Also numerically classified as MMP-16
- Chromosomal location: 8q 21.[30]
- Biological activity: MMP- 16 could transform pro- MMP 2 to activate MMP- 2 and thereby facilitate tumor invasion.[32]
- Group of substrates for enzymes: Collagen III, gelatine, casein.[30]

MT- MMP - 4

- Also numerically classified as MMP-17
- Chromosomal location: 12q 24.3.[30]
- Biological activity: It is expressed in a variety of human tissues mainly leukocyte colon, ovary, testis and the brain. The expression of MMP- 17 in leukocytes together with its membrane localization suggest that it could be involved in leukocytes together with its membrane location suggest that it could be involved in activation of membrane bound precursors of growth factors or inflammatory mediators such as TNF- α.[31,32]
- Group of substrates for enzymes: Collagen III, fibrinogen, proteoglycans.[30]

MT- MMP - 5

- Also numerically classified as MMP-24

- Chromosomal location: 20q 11.2.[30]

- Biological activity: It is essential modulator of neuroimmune interaction in thermal pain stimulation, and a mediator of peripheral thermal nociception and inflammatory hyperalgesia.[31,32]
- Group of substrates for enzymes: Proteoglycans.[30]

Review of Literature

Hong SD, et al. (2000),[40] did a study to compared MMP-2 and MMP-9 expression in 19 metastasizing oral SCCs with that in 25 non-metastasizing cases in order to evaluate the significance of matrix metalloproteinases (MMPs) in predicting the metastatic potential of oral squamous cell carcinomas (SCCs). The results revealed no significant difference in the activated form of MMP-2 between metastasizing and non- metastasizing oral SCCs. In metastasizing SCCs, on the other hand, increases in the activated form of MMP-9 were significant. These results suggest that oral SCCs express MMP-2 and MMP-9, and that MMP-9 may play a more important role than MMP-2 in the metastasis of oral SCCs to adjacent tissue. An analysis of MMP-9 expression may be useful for predicting the metastatic potential of oral SCCs.

Okuda K, et al. (2001),[41] evaluated the levels of tissue inhibitor of metalloproteinases- 1 (TIMP-1) and matrix metalloproteinases-1(MMP-1) and -8 (MMP-8) in gingival crevicular fluid following treatment with enamel matrix derivative. Sixteen patients with infrabony defects located contra laterally in the same arch, were included in this study. Patients were randomly assigned treatment with flap surgery plus EMD or flap surgery plus placebo. At baseline and at 2, 4 and 12 week follow-up evaluation visits, GCF was sampled with paper strips. At 4 weeks after surgery, GCF volume and TIMP- 1 levels showed a significant decrease in the EMD group. MMP-1 levels at weeks 2, 4 and 12, and MMP-8 levels at weeks 4 and 12 were significantly lower in the EMD group compared to the placebo group. These findings suggest that treatment with flap surgery and EMD, compared to flap surgery with placebo, accelerated healing at an earlier stage of wound healing following surgery.

T. Alpagot, et al. (2001),[42] did a study to evaluate GCF MMP-3 and TIMP-1 levels as prognostic factors for progressive periodontal disease. 40 medically healthy subjects were selected and clinical measurements including gingival index (GI), plaque index, bleeding on probing, suppuration, probing depth (PD), attachment loss (AL), and GCF samples were taken from 2 healthy sites and 2 periodontitis sites of each patient at baseline, 3-month and 6-month visits by means of sterile paper strips. The mean amounts of MMP-3 and TIMP-1 in diseased sites were significantly higher than in healthy sites. Significantly higher GCF levels of MMP-3 and TIMP-1 were found at progressing sites than in non-progressing periodontitis sites. These data indicate that sites with high GCF levels of MMP-3 and TIMP-1 are at significantly greater risk for progression of periodontitis.

Markus Kiili, et al. (2002), [43] did a study to determine the cellular and molecular forms of MMP-8 and MMP-13 associated with chronic adult periodontitis by examining the gingival crevicular fluid (GCF) and enzyme distribution in gingival tissues. GCF samples were collected directly from the periodontal pockets of 12 untreated patients using filter paper strips. After elution into buffer, the samples were examined by Western immunoblotting with polyclonal antibodies for MMP-8 and MMP-13 and quantification by scanning image analysis. The study concluded that multiple species and elevated levels of both MMP-8 and MMP-are identified in untreated periodontitis GCF and active forms contribute to GCF collagenase activity.

E Hrabec, et al. (2002),[44] investigated the expression and activation of MMP-2 and MMP-9 in lung cancer compared with normal lung parenchyma. Thirty-six pulmonary carcinomas and normal lung specimens were analyzed for the expression of MMP-2 and MMP-9. It was shown that expression of both MMP-2 and MMP-9 was remarkably higher in carcinoma samples than in normal lung specimen. The study concluded that

MMP-2 activation is associated with the malignant phenotype and may serve as a good marker of malignancy.

Kinane DF, et al. (2003),[45] did a study to investigate the effect of scaling and root planing (SRP) and the maintenance phase of treatment on the gingival crevicular fluid (GCF) matrix metalloproteinase-8 (MMP-8) levels. Clinical measurements and GCF samples were taken from four sites in 20 adult periodontitis patients before and after SRP and during a 3-month maintenance phase of treatment. MMP-8 levels were measured from GCF samples. Clinical improvement following SRP was associated with significant reductions in MMP-8 levels. The GCF concentration of MMP-8 decreased after initial therapy but reduced even more following a 3-month period of maintenance.

L Zhang, et al. (2004),[46] conducted a study to measure the expression of mRNAs and enzymatic activities of MMP-9 and -2 in prostate tissues and serum samples from men with or without prostate cancer. A total of 44 tissue samples and 71 serum samples were collected and the level of mRNA for MMP-2 and -9 was determined. Expression of MMP-9 mRNA was significantly higher in malignant than in nonmalignant prostate tissues. Results of zymography showed that there was significant difference in the enzymatic activity of MMP-9, but not MMP-2, among normal prostate, localized and metastatic prostate cancer tissues, serum samples. The study concluded that the activity of MMP-9 and the ratio of active form/proform of MMP-2 are associated with the progression and metastasis of prostate cancer.

M Pesta et al, (2005),[47] did a study to assess the levels of MMP-2, MMP-7, TIMP-1 and TIMP-2 mRNA expression in colorectal carcinoma tissue samples and to correlate them with the stage of the disease. The study included samples of tumor tissue of 38 patients with colorectal carcinoma and samples of tissue of 11 patients with benign disease. The levels of mRNA MMP-2, MMP-7, TIMP-1, TIMP-2 and glyceraldehyde- 3-phosphate dehydrogenase (GAPDH), as housekeeping gene, were quantified in tissue samples using the method of reverse transcription real-time PCR. The levels of mRNA expression of MMP-2, MMP-7 and TIMP-1 were found to be significantly higher in tumor tissue samples that in the control tissue.

Emingil G, et al. (2006),[48] did a study to examine the levels and molecular forms of MMP-7, tissue inhibitor of MMP (TIMP)-1, and extracellular matrix metalloproteinase inducer (EMMPRIN) in gingival crevicular fluid (GCF) from patients with different periodontal diseases. A total of 80 subjects 20 patients with generalized aggressive periodontitis, 20 with chronic periodontitis [CP], 20 with gingivitis, and 20 periodontally healthy subjects) were included in this study. It was concluded that MMP- 7 is associated with the innate host defense in periodontal tissues. Increased EMMPRIN and TIMP-1 levels in GCF are associated with the enhanced severity of periodontal inflammation, indicating that these molecules can participate in the regulation of progression of periodontal diseases.

Kumar MS, et al. (2006),[49] did a study to assess the expression of MMP-8 and MMP- 9 in gingival tissues of diabetic chronic periodontitis (CP), non-diabetic CP, and healthy patients.The levels of MMP expression in gingival tissue extracts were measured by gelatin zymography and Western blotting. The study found that the average concentration of MMP-9 was increased three-fold, and the MMP-8 was increased two- fold in CP patients with DM compared to CP patients without DM. An increased concentration of MMP-8 and -9 in the gingival tissue of diabetic CP patients suggests that the expression of these MMPs contributes to the failure of the healing process in the diabetic condition.

Ewa Kopczyńska, et al. (2007),[50] did a study to estimate effectiveness of MMP-9 activity in lung cancer patients, by serum MMP-9/TIMP-1 concentration ratio. The study group consisted of 49 patients with non-small-cell lung cancer. Serum concentration of MMP-9 and TIMP-1 was evaluated by ELISA. It was found that MMP-9 serum concentration and MMP-9/TIMP-1 ratio were significantly higher in IIIB-IV stage than I-IIIA, whereas TIMP-1 concentration did not show increasing tendency with tumour stage. The study concluded thatin later stages of lung cancer the balance between MMP-9 and TIMP-1 is altered, and MMP-9 activity is increased.

Rysz J, et al. (2007),[51] performed a study to access the levels of serum MMP-9, MMP- 2, TIMP-2 and TIMP-1in patients with diabetic neuropathy. Serum MMP-9, MMP-2, TIMP-2 and TIMP-1 were measured in patients with either chronic renal failure (CRF, n=20), type 2 diabetes mellitus (DM2, n=16), diabetic nephropathy (DM2+CRF, n=14), and healthy controls (n=20). It was found that diabetic nephropathy was related with profound decrease of serum TIMP-2, TIMP-1 and MMP-2. Both TIMP-1 and TIMP-2 were reduced in diabetic nephropathy in comparison with either diabetes alone or CRF alone. These data indicate that circulating TIMP-1, TIMP-2 and MMP-2 are decreased in patients with diabetic nephropathy when compared with either CRF or diabetes.

Gürkan A, et al. (2008),[52] did a study to investigate MMP-2, MMP-9 and MMP-12 gene polymorphisms in relation to susceptibility to severe chronic periodontitis (CP). Genomic DNA was obtained from peripheral blood of 87 severe CP patients and 107 periodontally healthy subjects. MMP-2 , MMP-9 and MMP −12 gene polymorphisms were genotyped by polymerase chain reaction and restriction fragment length polymorphism. Probing depth, clinical attachment loss, supragingival plaque accumulation and bleeding on probing were recorded. The results suggested that MMP- 2, MMP-9 and MMP-12 polymorphisms are not associated with susceptibility to severe CP. However, MMP-9 gene might be associated with decreased susceptibility to severe periodontitis.

Bıyıkoğlu B, et al. (2009),[53] did a study to compare gingival crevicular fluid (GCF) levels of matrix metalloproteinase (MMP)-8 and −13 and tissue inhibitor of MMP (TIMP)-1 in patients with rheumatoid arthritis (RA) and systemically healthy counterparts with inflammatory periodontal disease. 74 subjects were included and full- mouth clinical periodontal measurements were performed at six sites/tooth. GCF samples obtained from two sites in single-rooted teeth were analyzed. The total amounts of MMP-8 were lower in the healthy control group than in RA-gingivitis, RA- periodontitis, and healthy-periodontitis groups. Patients with RA and gingivitis or periodontitis exhibited levels of MMP-8 and −13 and TIMP-1 that were similar to systemically healthy counterparts. The study concluded that the coexistence of RA and periodontitis did not significantly affect the investigated parameters. GCF MMP-8 levels increased with periodontal inflammation.

Schumann C, et al. (2010),[54] tested the hypothesis that plasma concentration of matrix metalloproteinase (MMP)-2, tissue inhibitor of matrix metalloproteinases (TIMP)-4 and tenascin C (TNC) might be useful as biomarkers for assessing the severity of pulmonary hypertension (PH). Therefore, the concentrations of MMP-2, TIMP-4, TNC and N-terminal b-type natriuretic peptide (NT-proBNP) of 36 PH patients were compared with those of 44healthy volunteers.In PH patients, significantly elevated plasma levels of MMP-2, TIMP-4, TNC and NT-proBNP were detected. Monitoring of plasma TIMP-4, MMP-2 and TNC levels in PH patients might help to assess the beneficial effects of PH pharmacotherapy on tissue remodelling.

Rai B, et al. (2010),[55] conducted a study to determine the levels of GCF (gingival crevicular fluid) matrix metalloproteinase-8 (MMP-8) and metalloproteinase-9 (MMP- 9) patients with periodontitis and in healthy controls. Ten patients with periodontitis and ten healthy controls were included in the study. Levels of crevicular MMP-8 and - 9 were determined by ELISA in the subjects. Significantly higher crevicular MMP-8 and -9 were observed in cases of periodontitis compared to healthy adults.

A. Venkateshwari, et al. (2011),[56] did a study to evaluate the clinical significance of plasma concentration of MMP-9 in chronic pancreatitis. The samples were obtained from 112 chronic pancreatitis patients and healthy controls. MMP-9 levels were quantitatively measured by ELISA assay. The study revealed a significant increase of plasma MMP 9 levels in chronic pancreatitis patients compared to control subjects. Elevated levels were also observed in all the patient groups compared to control subjects. MMP-9 degrades the type IV collagens in normal basement membrane, which in turn activates the pancreatic stellate cells which promote the development of pancreatitic fibrosis. Thus, elevated plasma levels of MMP-9 may act as a susceptibility factor for the development of chronic pancreatitis.

Reddy NR, et al. (2012),[57] did a study to estimate the levels of MMP-3 in GCF in periodontal health, disease and to evaluate the effect of periodontal therapy on MMP-3 concentrations in GCF. Periodontal examination and collection of GCF by was performed in 30 subjects. Group I (Healthy, n= 10), group II (Chronic periodontitis, n= 20) and group III (After treatment group, n= 20). Scaling and root planing (SRP) was performed and GCF was collected after 8 weeks of treatment. MMP-3 levels were estimated in GCF samples.MMP-3 was detected in all samples. Highest mean MMP-3 concentrations in GCF were obtained for group II while the lowest concentrations were seen in group I and group III. This suggests that MMP-3 levels in GCF increases proportionally with the progression of periodontal disease and decreases after treatment.

Reddy NR, et al. (2014),[58] did a study to estimate tissue inhibitor of matrix metalloproteinase-1 (TIMP-1) levels in gingival crevicular fluid in periodontal health, disease and after treatment. Periodontal examination was done followed by GCF collection by extracrevicular method in 25 subjects categorized into three groups. Group I consisted of healthy patients, Group II consisted of patients with chronic periodontitis and Group III had patients with periodontitis after treatment. Scaling and root planning was performed and GCF was collected after 8 weeks of treatment. Highest mean TIMP-1 concentrations in GCF were obtained for Group I, whereas the lowest concentrations were seen in Group II. This suggests that TIMP-1 levels in GCF decreases proportionally with the progression of periodontal disease and increases after treatment.

Amato B, et al. (2015),[58] performed a study to evaluate the role of MMP-1 and MMP- 8 in long lasting and refractory venous ulcers. In a 2-year period 45 patients with chronic venous ulcers (CVU) were enrolled. The enrolled population was divided into two groups: group I were patients with non-healing ulcers and group II were patients with healing ulcers. MMP-1 and MMP-8 were measured in fluids and tissues of healing and non-healing ulcers by means of enzyme-linked immunosorbent assay (ELISA) and Western blot analysis, respectively. MMP-8 appeared in significantly greater amountsin the non-healing group. Our findings suggest that MMP-1, and MMP-8 are overexpressed in long lasting CVU.

Gupta N, et al. (2015),[59] investigated the role of salivary matrix metalloproteinase-8 (MMP-8) in chronic periodontitis diagnosis. The study included 20 healthy patients and
20 patients with chronic periodontitis. Around 3ml of unstimulated and whole expectorated saliva was collected for MMP-8 estimation. The results of this study demonstrate elevated concentrations of MMP-8 in individuals with chronic periodontitis.

Ebersole JL, et al. (2015),[60] conducted a study to evaluate the biomarkers representing various phases of periodontitis initiation and progression (IL-1ß, IL-6, MMP-8, MIP- 1α) in whole saliva from 209 subjects categorized with periodontal health, gingivitis, and periodontitis. Saliva samples were collected from the groups prior to clinical evaluation followed by a full mouth periodontal examination. IL-1β, IL-6, MMP-8 and MMP-1α concentrations were found to be significantly higher in the periodontitis group compared to levels in gingivitis and healthy subjects. The study showed that the salivary concentrations of IL-1ß, IL-6, MMP-8, MIP-1α alone and in combination are able to distinguish health from gingivitis and periodontitis.

Arreguin-Cano JA, et al. (2019),[61] did a study to evaluate MMP-2 salivary activity in type 2 diabetes mellitus patients. Ninety-seven type 2 diabetes mellitus patients were included in the study. Following clinical examination, the patients were classified into four groups according to the presence and degree of periodontal disease and glycemic control. Blood and whole saliva samples (WSS) were collected from each patient. Blood samples were used for Hba1c and polymorphonuclear cells count determination, while WSS were used to determine MMP-2 activity, TIMP-1 and nitrite. Salivary

MMP-2 activity, HbA1c and TIMP-1 were positively correlated with the severity of periodontitis. On the other hand, the increase in HbA1c was negatively correlated with MMP-2 activity and quantity of TIMP-1 but was positively correlated with nitrite levels.

Nardi GM, et al. (2020),[62] evaluated salivary Matrix Metalloproteinase (MMP-8) in periodontal patients undergoing non-surgical periodontal therapy along with mouthwash based on ozonated olive oil. Ninety-six subjects with a diagnosis of periodontitis were enrolled in this study and randomly assigned The study concluded that scaling and root planing with the aid of ozonated olive oil mouthwash were found to be more effective on salivary MMP-8 reduction than scaling and root planing alone.

Sioustis IA, et al. (2021),[63] did a study to identify the biomarkers that facilitate the assessment of periodontal status during orthodontic treatment. The study was conducted on 111 patients about to receive fixed orthodontic treatment. The salivary levels of MMP-8 and MMP-9 and bleeding on probing (BOP) before applying the orthodontic fixed appliance (T1), one week after appliance placement (T2), during orthodontic treatment, one month after non-surgical periodontal treatment (T3) were determined. The study patients undergoing orthodontic treatment showed a significant increase in BOP, MMP-8, and MMP-9 levels one week after orthodontic appliance placement and a decrease in these parameters was seen one month after periodontal treatment. Strong positive statistically significant correlations were found between MMP-8 levels and BOP and medium positive statistically significant correlations between MMP-9 and BOP values before and after orthodontic treatment and periodontal treatment. MMP-8, MMP-9, and BOP could be used to assess the periodontal status of orthodontic patients.

Structure of MMPs

Lovejoy et al. reported the first structure of MMP-inhibitor complex.[24] This structure reveals that the active site of MMP is a deep cavity and moreover that the catalytic domains of MMPs share a sequential similarity, where the percentage of similarity ranges between 33% (between MMP-21 and MMP23) and 86% (between MMP-3 and MMP-10). The most common structural features are: [64,31,65]

1- A signal N-terminal peptide with variable length, that targets the peptide for secretion;
2- A pro-domain (with about 80 aa), which keeps MMP inactive and is removed when the enzyme is proteolytically activated;
3- A catalytic domain (with about 160 aa), with a zinc ion, that consists of five β- sheets, three α-helixes and three calcium ions;
4- A linker of variable length (14–69 aa), which links the catalytic domain to hemopexin-like domain— "hinge region".
5- A hemopexin-like domain (with about 210 aa) that is characterized by four β- propeller.
6- An additional transmembrane domain with the small cytoplasmatic C-terminal domain, only present in MMPs-14, -15, -16 and -24.

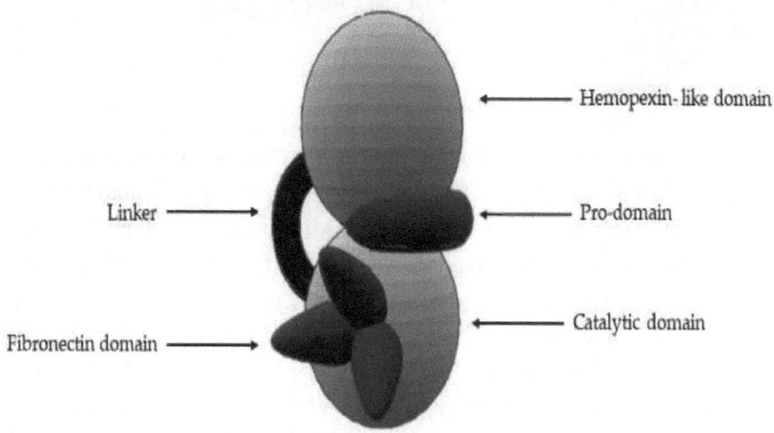

All MMPs are synthesized with an N-terminal signal sequence, which is removed in the endoplasmic reticulum, producing pro-enzymes. The pro-domain contains three α-helixes. In the case of MMP-1 and -2, the first loop has a cleavage region— "bait-region" —which is protease sensitive. The α(3)-helixes are followed by a "cysteine switch", a very conserved region (PRCGXPD), where the sulfhydryl group (Cys residue) coordinates the catalytic zinc forming a tetrahedral coordination sphere, thereby blocking enzyme.[65, 66,67]

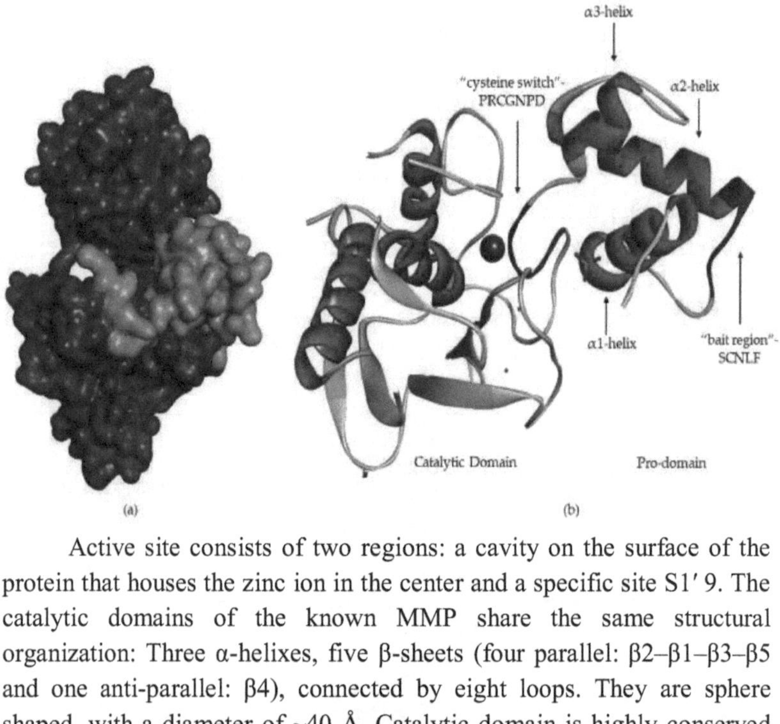

Active site consists of two regions: a cavity on the surface of the protein that houses the zinc ion in the center and a specific site S1′ 9. The catalytic domains of the known MMP share the same structural organization: Three α-helixes, five β-sheets (four parallel: β2–β1–β3–β5 and one anti-parallel: β4), connected by eight loops. They are sphere shaped, with a diameter of ~40 Å. Catalytic domain is highly conserved and in addition to catalytic zinc ions contain another Zn2+, that has a structural function, three calcium ions and three histidine residue that are part of a highly conserved sequence: VAAHEXGHXXGXXH. [66,67,68] The Ω-loop is found between α2-helix and α3-helix, its length and amino acid composition vary significantly among MMPs. This loop is the least conserved fragment within the catalytic domain, which is most likely responsible for different selectivity of MMPs.[68] In the terminal zone of the catalytic domain, located 8 residues down from the Zn2+, there is a region that forms the outer wall of pocket S1′ —"met-turn" (XBMX)[69]. The second zinc ion and the three calcium ions, that are present is all MMPs, have only a structural function and they been crucial for maintaining protein conformation.[70] Glutamic acid adjacent to the first histidine residue is essential for the catalytic process.[69, 71]

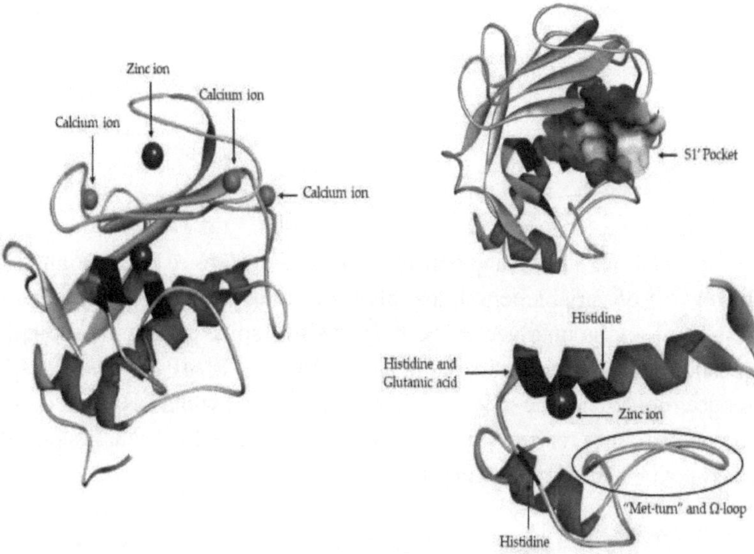

The hemopexin-like domain has four β-propeller structural elements. This domain is necessary for collagen triple helix degradation and is important for substrate specificity.[72] It also may be essential for the recognition and subsequent catalytic degradation of fibrillar collagen, whereas the catalytic domain is sufficient for the degradation of non-collagen substrates.[69] The only MMPs that don't have the hemopexin-like domain are MMP-7, -23, and -26. In the case MMP-23, this domain is substituted by an immunoglobulin-like domain and a cysteine-rich domain located immediately after the C-terminal of the catalytic domain.[73]

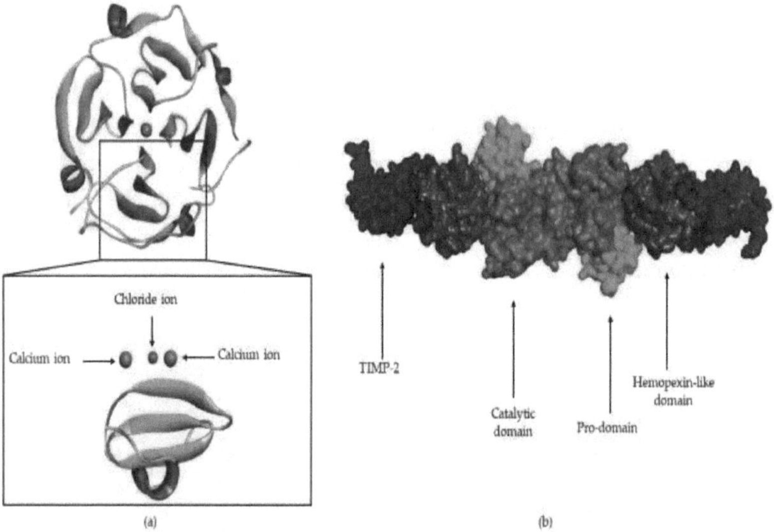

Catalytic and hemopexin-like domains are linked by a proline-rich linker [71,72] of variable length that allows inter-domain flexibility, enzyme stability[72] and is involved in the hydrolysis of some structurally complex substrates.[65] Mutations in the linker region in MMP-1[74] and MMP-8 reduce collagenolytic activity, supporting the hypothesis that correct movement and rearrangement between the catalytic domain and the hemopexin-like domain is important for activity.

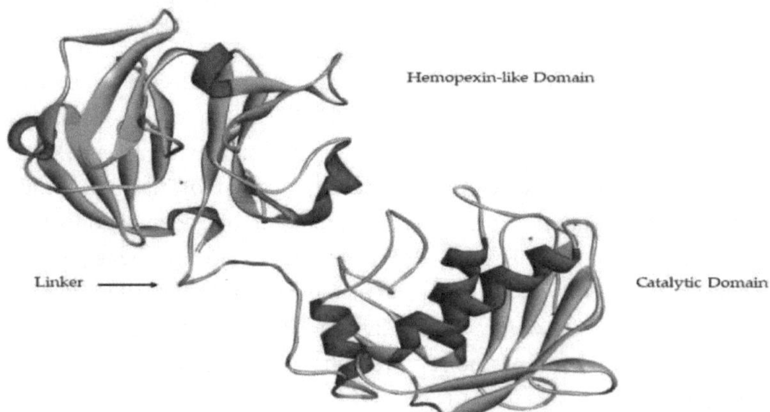

MMPs possess six pockets (S1, S2, S3, S1′, S2′, and S3′) [68] and the fragments of the substances and inhibitors are consequently named after the pocket that they interact with (P1, P2, P3, P1′, P2′, and P3′).[75] The S1, S2, and S3 pockets are unprimed pockets, which are localized on the right side of zinc ion. The S1′, S2′, and S3′ pockets are the primed pockets, which are localized on the left side of zinc ion.[68] It has been demonstrated that the S1′ is the most variable pocket in MMPs, followed by S2, S3′, S1, and S3 pockets with an equivalent degree of variance, while the S2′ has the lowest variability. The S2′ and S3′ pockets are shallower than S1′ and are more exposed to solvent. The S3 pocket may also contribute to substrate specificity.[69]

S1′ pocket is the most important since it is a determining factor for substrate specificity. Its cavity is formed by the Ω-loop is a highly hydrophobic. By analyzing the depth of the different S1′ subsites, MMPs can be divided into three different subgroups: the shallow, the intermedium and the deep pockets.[24,64]

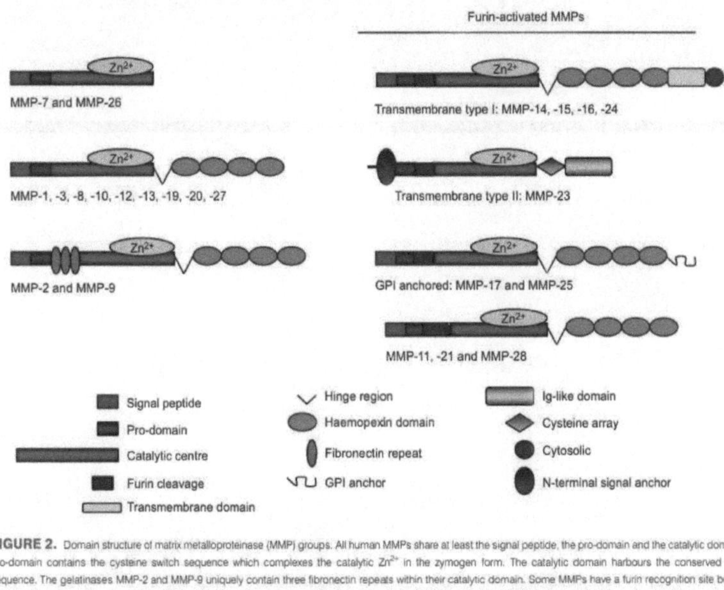

FIGURE 2. Domain structure of matrix metalloproteinase (MMP) groups. All human MMPs share at least the signal peptide, the pro-domain and the catalytic domain. The pro-domain contains the cysteine switch sequence which complexes the catalytic Zn^{2+} in the zymogen form. The catalytic domain harbours the conserved catalytic sequence. The gelatinases MMP-2 and MMP-9 uniquely contain three fibronectin repeats within their catalytic domain. Some MMPs have a furin recognition site before the catalytic domain, which allows intracellular activation of the zymogen by furin. Except for MMP-7 and -26, all MMPs have a flexible proline-rich hinge region and a haemopexin-like C-terminal domain, which function in substrate recognition. The membrane bound MMP-14, -15, -16, and -24 contain in addition a transmembrane and cytosolic domain, while MMP-17 and -25 are integrated in the plasma membrane by e glycosylphosphatidylinositol (GPI) anchor. Ig: immunoglobulin.

Activation of Pro-MMPs

MMPs are synthesized as pre-pro-MMPs, from which the signal peptide is removed during translation to generate pro-MMPs. In these zymogens or pro-MMPs, the cysteine from the PRCGXPD "cysteine-switch" motif coordinates with the catalytic Zn2+ to keep the pro-MMPs inactive MMPs can be activated by proteinases or in vitro by chemical agents.[76] Low pH and heat treatment can also lead to activation.[77] In order to process and activate these zymogens or pro-MMPs, the cysteine switch is cleaved and the prodomain is detached often by other proteolytic enzymes such as serine proteases, the endopeptidase furin, plasmin, or other MMPs to produce the active MMP forms.[76] Furin-containing MMPs such as MMP-11, -21, and -28, and MT-MMPs have a furin-like pro-protein convertase recognition sequence at the C-terminus of the propeptide and are activated intracellularly by furin.[78] MT-MMPs first undergo intracellular activation by furin, then proceed to the cell surface where they can cleave and activate other pro-MMPs.[79] TIMPs are also essential for the formation of noninhibitory pro-MMP/TIMP/MT-MMP complexes. Noninhibitory complexes between progelatinases and TIMPs are restricted to pro-MMP-2 and TIMP-2, -3, or -4, and to MMP-9 and TIMP-1.[80] For example, TIMP-2 first forms a complex with pro- MMP-2 by binding to its hemopexin domain, and the complex then localizes to the cell surface where it binds to the active site of a MT1-MMP molecule.[81,82] This ternary pro- MMP-2/TIMP-2/MT1–MMP complex then facilitates the cleavage and activation of its bound pro-MMP-2 to active MMP-2 by another "free" MT1-MMP molecule. This noninhibitory complex is different from the inhibitory complex of TIMP-2/active MMP-2. It is formed between the C-terminal domain of TIMP-2 and the C-terminal hemopexin of MMP-2, such that both molecules maintain their inhibitory and proteolytic properties, respectively.[83,84] The activation of MMP-2 on the cell surface allows it to accumulate pericellularly where it could reach marked collagenolytic activity locally in the extracellular space. Similarly, the stromelysins MMP-3 and -10 are secreted from the cells as inactive pro- 9MMPs, but are then activated on the cell surface. MMPs can also be activated by various physicochemical agents including heat, low pH, thiol-modifying agents such as 4-aminophenylmercuric acetate, mercury chloride, N-ethylmaleimide, oxidized glutathione, sodium dodecyl sulfate, and chaotropic agents. Most of these activators disrupt the cysteine-$Zn2+$ coordination at the cysteine-switch motif of the MMP molecule. Other MMP activators include plasmin which activates MMP-9. Also, both MMP-3 and hypochlorous acid activate MMP-7, and MMP-7 could in turn activate MMP-1.[85] MMP expression can also be influenced by hormones, growth factors, and cytokines.[71] For example, ovarian sex hormones could affect the expression/activity of various MMPs which could in turn participate in endometrial tissue remodeling and shedding during the menstrual and estrous cycles. Also, increases in estrogen and progesterone as well as vascular endothelial growth factor (VEGF) and placental growth factor during pregnancy could promote the expression/activity of uteroplacental MMPs and in turn facilitate cytotrophoblast tissue invasion and uteroplacental growth and vascularization. MMP expression/activity also increases during the inflammatory process. MMPs are secreted by proinflammatory cells and their secretion is promoted by proinflammatory cytokines. MMPs can be regulated by growth factors.[86] For example, overexpression of VEGFa in SNU-5 cells increases MMP-2 expression, while downregulation of VEGFa decreases MMP-2 expression.[87] Also, platelet derived growth factor-BB (PDGF-BB) increases MMP-2 expression in rat VSMCs, possibly via Rho-associated protein kinase, extracellular signal-regulated kinases (ERK), and phosphorylation of p38 mitogenactivated protein kinase (MAPK).[88] Also, in carotid artery plaques, epidermal growth factor (EGF) upregulates MMP-1 and -9 mRNA transcripts and increases MMP-9 activity in

VSMCs. In contrast, transforming growth factor-β1 (TGF-β1) may downregulate MMPs via a TGF-β1 inhibitory element in the MMP promoter. Interestingly, MMP-2 does not have this element, and therefore may not be affected, or in some instances upregulated, by TGF-β1. MMP activity is also regulated by endogenous TIMPs. Increased MMP expression/activity or decreased TIMPs could lead to MMP/TIMP imbalance and results in various pathological conditions most notably heart failure, osteoarthritis, and cancer.[89]

Physiologic Functions of MMPs

MMPS IN BONE MODELLING AND REMODELLING

Bone is an important site of ongoing tissue remodelling during development, homeostasis and repair. Bone develops according to one of three distinct processes: intramembranous ossification, endochondral ossification or pseudo-metamorphic ossification.[90] Loss of MMP9 is associated with growth-plate defects. The first developmental phenotype reported in an MMP knockout mouse was a defect in endochondral ossification of long bones. Deletion of Mmp9 results in expansion of the zone of hypertrophic chondrocytes in the growth plate because of a failure of apoptosis.[91] A relevant MMP9 substrate seems to be galectin-3, a lectin with antiapoptotic activity that can be secreted and localized to the ECM. MMP9 cleaves and inactivates galectin-3. Indeed, galectin-3-mutant mice display growth-plate defects that are opposite of the defects of Mmp9-deficient mice, with premature apoptosis of the hypertrophic chondrocytes.[92] Uncleaved galectin-3 is also enriched specifically at the growth plate in Mmp9 mutants. MMP9 is also highly expressed during bone healing after fracture, and bone fractures in Mmp9-mutant mice heal more slowly than in controls. Exogenous vascular endothelial growth factor (VEGF) rescues the repair defects, indicating that MMP9 processing of VEGF might be rate limiting in bone repair.[93] MMP13 functions in bone formation and remodelling. Mmp13 mutants show an expansion of the zone of hypertrophic chondrocytes and a delay in apoptosis, indicating that MMP13 is required for the transition from cartilage to bone at the growth plates of long bones.[94] MMP13 cleaves type II collagen and aggrecan in vivo, and these cleavage products can be recognized in a tight zone that is just distal to the zone of ossification and angiogenesis. The primary defect in Mmp13 mutants is a failure of chondrocytes to remodel the ECM that is rich in type II collagen and aggrecan. Collagen cleavage does not occur in the absence of MMP13, whereas both MMP13 and MMP9 cleave aggrecan. The second function of MMP13 in long-bone development occurs during ossification. The cartilage ECM becomes the scaffold for mineralization, forming bone spicules or trabeculae. Mmp13 mutants exhibit irregularly shaped spicules, demonstrating that MMP13 is required for their initial modelling.[95]

MMP IN BLOOD VESSEL REMODELLING

Analysis of a broad range of MMP mutants shows that embryonic vascular development proceeds normally, yet defects are observed in both normal and pathological postnatal vascular remodelling and angiogenesis. MMPs might have a specific role in postnatal refinement, remodelling and neoangiogenesis, but not in the original construction of the embryonic vascular networks. Mmp9-mutant mice show defects in angiogenesis at the growth plate of long bones.[91] Similarly, Mmp14-mutant mice lack appropriate vascular invasion at secondary ossification centres, despite normal levels of VEGF and its receptor VEGFR2.[96] Likely mechanisms include proteolysis of type I collagen, modification of platelet-derived growth factor (PDGF) signalling, regulation of perivascular cells and processing of VEGF. Invading blood vessels in post natal tissues encounter ECM that is rich in type I collagen, a protein that is not highly expressed in embryos. When control aortic explants are embedded in three-dimensional collagen matrices, they sprout neovessels and the endothelial cells invade the collagen matrix in a growth factor-dependent manner.[97] MMP9 and MMP14 have another effect on the vasculature: the perivascular (or smooth muscle) cells that ensheath the endothelial cells of the blood vessels are missing or their density is significantly decreased in normal vessels and during tumour neoangiogenesis. [98]

MMPS IN INFLAMMATION AND WOUNDING

The role of MMPs is not limited to developmental processes, and mouse-mutant experiments are beginning to show that MMPs are also required to maintain homeostasis in response to environmental challenges, such as wounding and infection.[99] MMP7 is involved in innate immunity and wound healing. MMP7 (or matrilysin) has no known role in development and is not expressed at high levels in embryonic development. In healthy adult tissue, MMP7 is expressed only in mucosal epithelia and it is upregulated and proteolytically activated in response to bacterial exposure in epithelia.[100] MMP7 is also required for wound healing. MMP7 seems to mediate wound-induced epithelial migration by cleaving E-cadherin.[101] MMP7 co localizes with E-cadherin and cleaves its extracellular domain in wounded epithelia, which results in a loosening of cell–cell attachments. Both injury and infection induce inflammation, another physiological response to environmental challenge that requires MMPs. MMPs facilitate inflammatory cell recruitment and clearance of inflammatory cells by cleaving inflammatory mediators, resulting in a tightly regulated inflammatory response.[102-104] Several chemokines, including C–C motif ligand-7 (CCL7) and CXCL12, are substrates for MMP2. MMP9 cleaves and activates CXCL6 and CXCL8 (also known as interleukin-8 , whereas it inactivates CXCL1 and CXCL4.[105]

MMPs in the Pathogenesis of Periodontal Disease

Inflammatory destruction of periodontal attachment apparatus is the hallmark of periodontal disease, and degradation of type I collagen seen in periodontal tissues is a key step in periodontal attachment loss. Degradation action on collagen fibers is performed by MMPs released by the resident cells of PDL that responds to the inflammatory stimuli. The most common type of MMPs related to tissue destruction belongs to collagenases family and includes mainly MMP-8 and MMP-13, with significant contribution from MMP-9 and MMP-14.[106]

Majority of the studies performed on the role of this group of MMPs have studied the effects of subtype 8 and 13 in periodontitis. MMP-8 has the unique ability to break down the type I and III collagen which is critical for periodontal destruction. Increased salivary MMP-8 levels were found in periodontitis and gingivitis patients with significant correlation with clinical parameters, which could be attributed to the ability of MMP-8 to degrade type I and III collagen necessary for periodontal destruction.[107] Neutrophils are the major cellular sources of MMP-8, and a large persistent neutrophil influx is seen in periodontal diseases.[108] It has been found that the neutrophil collagenase activity in GCF of patients with periodontitis and concluded that collagenase activity was positively associated with the severity of periodontal disease and MMP-8 accounted for most of the activity. MMP-1 and MMP-13 may be associated with tissue remodelling in chronic wounds and thus could be used as potential markers of repair in diseased periodontal tissues.[109] Marcaccini et al (2009) have demonstrated increased levels of MMP-8 in patients with chronic periodontitis than in controls with decreased levels 3 months after therapy and moderate correlation with clinical parameters. They also reported increased plasma levels of MMP-8 and MMP-9 in patients with chronic periodontitis and emphasized the importance of periodontal therapy to avoid elevated levels, which are associated with many systemic disorders.[110]

MMP-8 levels have been found to be significantly higher in chronic periodontitis, and scaling and root planning has found to significantly reduce MMP-8 levels 4 weeks after therapy although the levels did not reduce to normal values. Increased salivary MMP- 8 concentration in periodontitis subjects than in controls could be used as valuable marker for the detection of periodontitis .[111]

Matrix metalloproteinase-2 and MMP-9 belong to this family of metalloproteinases. MMP-2 is secreted by gingival fibroblasts, and MMP-9 is mainly secreted by PMLs and they degrade collagen type IV present in gingival tissues. Rai et al (2008) showed that crevicular MMP-9 levels were higher in periodontitis than in healthy controls, while the reverse was true for MMP-2 and the levels highly correlated with clinical attachment loss and bleeding on probing. Similar findings were also seen in several other studies.[112, 113] Ozcaka et al (2011) demonstrated that smokers with chronic periodontitis and smoking controls exhibited significantly higher serum concentration of MMP-9 than non-smoker counterpart.[108] Increased salivary and serum concentrations of MMP-2 and MMP-9 and decrease after periodontal therapy were demonstrated in several other studies implicating their role in periodontal diseases.[110] MMP-2 and MMP-9 were suggested to participate in tissue destruction and periodontitis.[112]

GCF levels of MMPs in patients with periodontitis were also studied in terms of their diagnostic and prognostic values. GCF levels of MMP-9 and -13 were suggested as useful biomarkers for periodontitis progression when active sites were defined in moderate to advanced chronic periodontitis patients followed for 2 months.[113] Another cross-sectional study reported that GCF MMPs-8 and -9 levels are correlated with disease activity in chronic periodontitis patients.[114] Higher levels of

MMP-3, -8, -9, and gelatinolytic activities have been reported in plasma of chronic periodontitis patients that decreased significantly 3 months after nonsurgical periodontal treatment.[115] Persistent elevation of MMP-8 in GCF samples is regarded as indicating high risk and poor response to periodontal therapy.[116] Furthermore, a chair- side MMP-8 test was indicated to effectively differentiate clinically healthy sites and gingivitis from chronic periodontitis and also effectively monitor the treatment of chronic periodontitis patients.[117]

As for bone resorption, MMP-9 is likely the most important proteinase involved in this process, as osteoclasts express this enzyme at high levels.[118] However, there are contradictory reports about the specific role of MMP-9 in bone resorption. For example, certain authors have suggested that MMPs make, at best, a very small contribution to the bone-resorptive activity of osteoclasts and that the selective inhibitor of MMP-9, TIMP-1, did not show a significant inhibitory effect on osteoclastic bone resorption, while other studies have reported that MMP-9 might play an essential role in the bone resorption caused by osteoclasts and that patients with MMP-9 genotypes, in association with their soluble protein, may have an increased risk of developing chronic periodontitis .[119] Previous studies have also shown that MMPs are present in peri-implant sulcular fluid and can play a pathologic role in peri-implant bone loss. MMP-8 has been reported to be present in peri-implant sulcular fluid. The polymorphism in the promoter of the MMP-8 gene could be a risk factor for early implant failure.[120, 121]

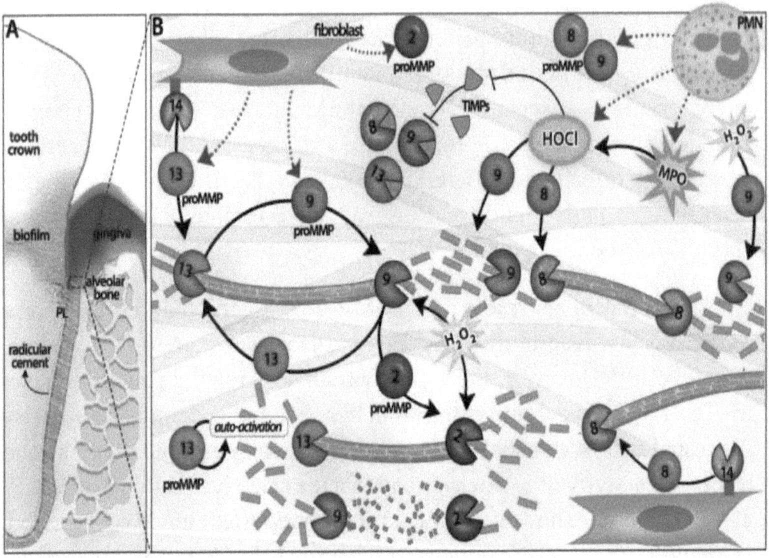

Figure 1. Matrix metalloproteinase (MMP) activation cascades in connective tissue catabolism during periodontitis. Full and partial circles with their respective number represent latent and activated specific MMPs. Brown T bars represent collagen fibers. (**A**) Tooth and its supporting structures: radicular cement, periodontal ligament (PL) and alveolar bone; (**B**) Membrane bounded MMP-14 activates proMMP-13 to degrade type I collagen, which constitutes the bulk component of radicular cement, periodontal ligament (PL) and alveolar bone extracellular matrix; MMP-13 activates proMMP-9, which in turn might activate proMMP-2 and proMMP-13. MMP-2 and MMP-9 further process gelatin resulting from collagenase activity. MMP-13 can undergo auto-activation by self-proteolysis. Reactive oxygen species, such as HOCl and H_2O_2, from phagocytes can also modify the proteases/anti-proteases balance, activating latent MMPs and inactivating the tissue inhibitor of MMPs (TIMP)-1. MPO, myeloperoxidase.

Inhibitors of MMPs

Endogenous inhibitors

A major group of inhibitors of MMPs are the tissue inhibitors of metalloproteinases (TIMPs). The four human TIMPs are the natural endogenous inhibitors of the matrix metalloproteinases (MMPs), a family of endopeptidases that regulate the turnover of extracellular matrix (ECM) and cleave various bioactive molecules including cytokines, chemokines and growth factors.[66] Tissue inhibitor of metalloproteinases (TIMP-1) was discovered in 1975 in form of a collagenase inhibitor present in human serum being released from skin fibroblasts.[122] TIMP-I, also known as TIMP, is a 30-kDa glycoprotein and is synthesized and secreted by most connective tissue cells as well as by macrophages. It also resides in platelet α granules and can be identified in most body fluids.[4] TIMP-2 is secreted by human melanoma cells and has similar inhibitory properties to TIMP-I, with a related but different sequence and may be controlled differently.[123,124] The third member of the family, TIMP-3, was first isolated in the chick. It has the unusual property of being found almost exclusively bound to the extracellular matrix.[125] The expression of MMPs and TIMPs by connective tissue cells in culture is regulated by a number of cytokines (particularly IL- l), growth factors and hormones. Many factors are the products of monocytes/macrophages and their production in inflammatory situations is a key step in initiating tissue degradation. TGF-/3 may be especially important since it can modulate the cytokine-induced synthesis of MMPs and TIMP.[126] The role of TIMPs may be to tightly control MMP activity both at the level of activation and subsequent substrate degradation. As with other proteinase-inhibitor systems (notably the well documented plasminogen activators) MMPs may be active only at specific locations where inhibitor concentrations compared with enzymes are reduced.[66]

TIMPs are specific inhibitors that bind MMPs in a 1:1 stoichiometry. Under pathological conditions associated with unbalanced MMP activities, changes of TIMP levels are considered to be important because they directly affect the level of MMP activity. TIMPs (21 to 29 kDa) have an N- and C-terminal domain of 125 and 65 amino acids, respectively, with each containing three conserved disulfide bonds.[127] The N- terminal domain folds as a separate unit and is capable of inhibiting MMPs. The N- terminal domain folds as a separate unit and is capable of inhibiting MMPs.[128] NMR first solved the structure of the N-terminal domain of TIMP-2 in 1994. The complete structure of TIMP-1 and of the inhibition mechanism was determined by X-ray crystallographic studies of the TIMP-1–MMP-3 complex, and soon after, that of the TIMP-2–MT1-MMP complex was determined. The overall shape of the TIMP molecule is like a wedge, which slots into the active-site cleft of an MMP in a manner similar to that of the substrate. Figure 5 shows the structures of the MT1-MMP catalytic domain, TIMP-2, and their interaction.[129] The main sites of interaction of TIMP-2 with the catalytic domain are the N-terminal four residues and the CD-loop region adjacent to them. The N-terminal four residues bind in the catalytic site cleft, making backbone contacts similar to those of a substrate. Residues at 1 and 3 are strictly conserved cysteines that form disulfide bonds in the main body of the protein. Cys1 is instrumental in chelating the active-site zinc with its N-terminal -amino group and carbonyl group, thereby expelling the water molecule bound to the catalytic zinc.[130]

The expression of MMPs and TIMPs by connective tissue cells in culture is regulated by a number of cytokines (particularly IL- l), growth factors and hormones, some of which are specific to cell type and others that are more ubiquitous (eg TGF-P). Many factors are the products of monocytes/macrophages and their production in inflammatory situations is a key step in initiating tissue degradation.[131] TGF-β may be especially important since it can modulate the cytokine-induced synthesis of MMPs (down) and TIMP.[132] Interaction between different factors is important when considering cells in tissues in vivo rather than in artificial culture models. Most cells synthesize TIMPs, yet little is known about the normal control of their levels in vivo, although activity is elevated by treating cells in vitro with phorbol esters, corticosteroids, TGF-P, fibroblast growth factor (FGF), retinoids and IL-1. Recent work has also implicated an important role for IL-11 in stimulating TIMP in human chondrocytes and synoviocytes. Preliminary studies suggest that TIMP-3 modulation may be different to that of TIMP-1.[133]

Exogenous inhibitors

$Zn2^{1}$- and $Ca2^{1}$-chelating agents (EDTA and 1,10- phenanthroline) are potent inhibitors of enzyme activity in vitro, but they are toxic and not used in vivo as therapeutic agents.[134] Multiple synthetic peptides have been formulated in an attempt to synthesize more specific chelators including phosphorus containing peptides, sulfur- based inhibitors and peptidyl hydroxamic acid derivatives. Phosphorus containing peptides are potent inhibitors of metalloproteinases produced by the substitution of a tetrahedral phosphorus atom for the carbonyl carbon atom in a peptide substrate. Phosphonamidate and phosphinate analogs of tripeptides can inhibit human skin fibroblast collagenase in vitro.[135] Sulfur based inhibitors of the matrix metalloproteinases were prepared by replacing the scissile C(½0)NH bond of the peptide with various sulfur-containing functional groups. The mercaptan derivatives were the most potent inhibitors of collagenases, gelatinases and stromelysin compared with all other sulfur- based inhibitors of matrix metalloproteinases in vitro.[136] Perhaps the most widely used synthetic peptides, and the ones receiving the most attention as potential pharmaceutical agents, are the hydroxamic acid derivatives. These are prepared by adding a hydroxamic acid residue at the C-terminus of the peptide as a metal-chelating moiety.[137] The hydroxamate group of these derivatives binds to the Zn^{2+} at the active site by two oxygen atoms, which together with three histidines makes the zinc pentacoordinated.[138] Hydroxamic acid derivatives are capable of inhibiting matrix metalloproteinases 1, 2, 3, 7, 8 and 9 in vitro with very low levels at which collagenase activity declines by 50% (such as the low nM range).[137] Several major pharmaceutical companies have generated a number of hydroxamic acid-type matrix metalloproteinase inhibitors and these are discussed below. Polyclonal and monoclonal antibodies have been synthesized in an attempt to discriminate between the closely related matrix metalloproteinase enzymes. Most recently bisphosphonates, primarily designed to modulate osteoclast function and not specifically designed to be matrix metalloproteinase inhibitors, have been found to inhibit matrix metalloproteinases 1, 3, 8 and 13 in vitro; the mechanism of action may involve cation chelation.[139]

Although a number of matrix metalloproteinase inhibitors have been developed over the past decade, only a few have been found to be safe and effective, particularly after oral administration. The tetracycline analogues are currently the only matrix metalloproteinase inhibitors approved by the US Food and Drug Administration being used clinically and, as discussed below, are the only proteinase inhibitors that have been clinically tested in humans for efficacy in periodontal therapy. Minocycline provided the first evidence of MMP inhibition by tetracycline (TC) and its derivatives in the oral environment, as it was observed to inhibit the collagenolytic activity of gingival cervicular fluid in the absence of bacteria.[140] TCs are antibiotics with cationic chelating properties that inhibit MMP activity in the extracellular environment and prevent proMMP activation through oxidation by scavenging reactive oxygen species. TCs down-regulate transcriptional MMP levels at the intracellular level.[141,142] Doxycycline hyclate is a low-dose tetracycline analogue deprived of antimicrobial activity and is indicated for the treatment of periodontal diseases, acting through the inhibition of MMP-8 and MMP-13 protease mechanisms. The therapeutic effect of this antibiotic is due to the modulation of the host response since the low-dose formulations have lost their antimicrobial activity. Tetracyclines are found to inhibit MMP activity by cationic binding proteins. The use of this drug in association with mechanical periodontal therapy has been widely accepted. In adults with periodontitis, low-dose doxycycline is currently used as an adjuvant therapy to inhibit MMP activity since it significantly reduces the severity of periodontal disease, including alveolar bone loss.[143] Chemically modified tetracyclines (CMTs) lack the 4-dimethylamino group of TCs, which exerts antibacterial activity. Several CMTs with a range of potency and specificity for MMP inhibition have been developed. CMTs-3 and -8 are the most potent inhibitors of MMPs, especially collagenases, and CMT-3 is the only CMT with demonstrated potency against MMP-1.[144]

Discussion

COLLAGENASES:

Collagenases include MMP-1 (interstitial collagenase), MMP-8 (neutrophil collagenase), MMP -13, and MMP-18. These MMPs play an important role in cleaving fibrillar collagen type I, II, and III. They first unwind triple-helical collagen, then hydrolyze the peptide bonds.[145]

MMP-1:

MMP-1, also termed collagenase-1 or interstitial collagenase. MMP-1 degrades collagen and gelatin. MMP-1 also cleaves pro-MMP-9 into its active form. As with many other MMPs, the levels of MMP-1 are very low in most cells under physiological conditions, but are upregulated in inflammatory conditions and autoimmune disease.[146] MMP-1 expression is augmented by inflammatory cytokines such as tumor necrosis factor-α (TNF-α) and interleukin-1 (IL-1). Increased levels and activities of MMP-1, - 8, and -9 with relatively low levels of TIMP have been identified in slow-to-heal wounds and venous wounds.[147] In cultured human vocal fold fibroblasts, TNF-α inhibits cell proliferation, downregulates TIMP-3 and the mRNA transcript levels for collagen III and fibronectin, and upregulates MMP-1 and -2 expression, resulting in increased MMP/TIMP-3 ratio, which may accelerate wound healing following vocal fold injury.[148] MMP-1 may play a role in cancer development and metastasis. Studies have suggested an association between SNP of MMP-1- 1607 2G/2G and poor prognosis in malignant tumors such as tongue squamous cell carcinoma. Also, in patients with invasive well-differentiated thyroid carcinoma, MMP-1 expression correlates with tumor aggressiveness manifested as laryngotracheal invasion, multi- focality of the tumor, and the presence of metastases. MMP-1 expression is associated with poor prognosis in esophageal cancer and may serve as a prognostic marker and an indicator for the need for more aggressive surgical intervention.[149,150]

MMP-8:

MMP-8, also termed collagenase-2 or neutrophil collagenase was discovered in cDNA library constructed from mRNA that was extracted from peripheral leukocytes of a patient with chronic granulocytic leukemia. Being a collagenase, MMP-8 can cleave interstitial collagens I, II, and III.[151] While some pro-MMPs are secreted then form heterodimeric complexes bound to TIMPs, secreted pro- MMP-8 remains in its free form. The pro-MMP-8 activity is then regulated by proteolytic cleavage by other MMPs such as MMP-3 and -10.[152] MMP-8 is the first collagenase to appear during dermal wound healing and its levels peak earlier than that of MMP-1, supporting time- dependent expression of different MMPs during wound healing.[153] Mice deficient in MMP-8 show delayed healing of cutaneous wounds and increased inflammatory responses, supporting that MMP-8 is a necessary component in dermal wound healing and the regulation of the inflammatory process.[154] In a study to assess the temporal relationship between periodontal tissue destruction and activity of collagenase, exudate from inflamed periodontal tissues was collected, and latent and active collagenase activities were measured It was found that the collagenase activity was derived from neutrophils, and there was an overall 40% increase of pooled active collagenase activity in all subjects with progressive loss of connective tissue. These findings suggest a role of neutrophil collagenase or MMP-8 in the destruction of periodontal connective tissue, and MMP-8 expression in the saliva may be used as a marker of diseases involving connective tissue breakdown and advanced periodontitis.[155]

MMP-13

MMP-13 is also termed collagenase-3. It is very efficient in degrading type II collagen. MMP- 13 was first thought to be expressed in connective tissue particularly cartilage and developing bone. However, MMP-13 has also been detected in epithelial and neuronal cells.[156] In comparison with normal cartilage, osteoarthritis cartilage shows an increased MMP-13 expression which may be associated to ECM remodelling in human chondrocytes. Thus MMP-13 may be a therapeutic target in treatment of osteoarthritis.[157] MMP-13 may be involved in lung diseases such as acute lung injury, viral infections, and chronic obstructive pulmonary disease. MMP-13 is involved in the secretion of these virus-induced proinflammatory chemokines. These observations support that MMP-13 plays a role in defense mechanisms of airway epithelial cells.[158] MMP-13 may be involved in ECM degradation in brain astrocytes. Conditioned medium collected from activated microglia increased IL-18 production and enhanced MMP-13 expression in astrocytes. Recombinant IL-18 stimulation also increased the enzymatic activity of MMP-13 and the migratory activity of. These findings suggest that IL-18 is an important regulator of MMP-13 expression and cell migration in astrocytes.[159] MMP-13 is often overexpressed in tumours and may increase the risk of tumour progression and metastasis. MMP-13 is overexpressed in nasopharyngeal cancer cells and exosomes purified from conditioned medium, as well as plasma of nasopharyngeal cancer patients. Tran swell analysis revealed that MMP-13-containing exosomes facilitated the metastasis of nasopharyngeal cancer cells.[160]

GELATINASES

Gelatinases include gelatinase A (MMP-2) and gelatinase B (MMP-9). MMP-2 and -9 are structurally similar to other proteinases in the MMP family, but differ in that they have a distinct collagen-binding domain composed of three fibronectin type II tandem repeats in the N-terminus of the catalytic domain, which is needed for gelatin binding. MMP-2 and -9 have been recognized as major contributors to proteolytic degradation of ECM. A number of nonmatrix proteins have been identified as gelatinase substrates. Thus these enzymes are proteolytic regulators in various physiological and pathological states including embryonic growth and development, angiogenesis, vascular diseases, inflammation, infective diseases, and degenerative diseases of the brain and tumor progression. MMP-2 and MMP-9 are particularly involved in cancer invasion and metastasis. [161,162]

MMP-2

MMP-2, also termed gelatinase A or type IV collagenase, cleaves collagen in two phases. The first resembling that of interstitial collagenase, followed by gelatinolysis. The collagenolytic activity of MMP-2 is much weaker than collagenases. However, pro-MMP-2 is recruited to the cell surface and undergoes autocatalytic cleavage. It therefore accumulates pericellularly and causes marked local collagenolytic activity.[163] MMP-2 is involved in a variety of physiological and pathological processes, including angiogenesis, tissue repair, and inflammation. MMP-2 and its inhibitors TIMP-1 and -2, also play a role in tumor invasion and metastasis, and MMP-2/TIMPs imbalance may contribute to tumor progression. MMP-2 activity was correlated with lymph node metastasis, and lymphatic and vascular invasion, supporting an important role of MMP-2 in the invasion of esophageal carcinoma.[164] MMP-2 levels also correlate with invasiveness of cancer cells and shortened survival independent of major prognostic indicators in patients with primary breast carcinoma. MMP-2 may also play a role in malignant tumors of the central nervous system.[165]

MMP-9

MMP-9 is produced by a variety of cells including epithelial cells, fibroblasts, keratinocytes, osteoblasts, dendritic cells, macrophages, granulocytes, and T-cells. MMP-9 plays a key role in inflammatory cell migration and in the destructive behavior of cholesteatoma. However, serum levels of MMP-9 might not correctly reflect the extent of localized tissue inflammation. In a study of patients with cholesteatoma, MMP-9 and TIMP-1 serum levels were similar with those in control group. In contrast, the levels of MMP-9 and TIMP-1 were higher in cholesteatoma tissues than normal skin specimens. These findings suggest better clinical usefulness of MMP-9 and TIMP- 1 expression in cholesteatoma tissues than either serum or plasma levels of these proteins and that the higher the expression of MMP-9 the stronger the inflammation- accompanied cholesteatoma.[166] MMP-9 is also expressed in migrating macrophages.[167] MMP-9 has also been detected in esophageal cancer and gelatin zymography showed a correlation between MMP-9 activity and vascular invasion of esophageal carcinoma.[168]

Stromelysins

Stromelysins 1, 2, and 3, also known as MMP-3, -10, and -11, respectively, have the same domain arrangement as collagenases, but do not cleave interstitial collagen. MMP-3 and -10 are similar in structure and substrate specificity, while MMP-11 is distantly related. MMP-3 and MMP-10 digest a number of ECM molecules and participate in pro-MMP activation, but MMP-11 has very weak activity toward ECM molecules. Also, MMP-3 and -10 are secreted from the cells as inactive pro-MMP, but MMP-11 is activated intracellularly by furin and secreted from the cells as an active enzyme.[169]

MMP-3

MMP-3, also known as stromelysin- possesses some unique characteristics. First, MMP-3 retains protease capability even if the zinc moiety is replaced with cobalt, manganese, cadmium, or nickel ions, but depending on the moiety, the protease activity becomes sensitive to different substrates. Second, MMP-3 has a unique deep active site that transverses the length of the enzyme.[170] MMP-3 is well known as a secretory endopeptidase that degrades ECM.109 MMP-3 preferentially cleaves proteins at sites where the first three amino acids following the cleavage site are hydrophobic.[171] MMP- 3 degrades collagen type II, IV, and IX as well as a variety of proteoglycans, elastin, fibronectin, and laminin. MMP-3 may activate other MMPs necessary for tissue remodelling including MMP-1, -7, and -9.[170] MMP-3 has been detected in the nucleus, and human nuclear MMP-3 may function as a trans-regulator of connective tissue growth factor. MMP-3 has also been detected in the nuclei of hepatocytes and may be involved in apoptosis. Heterochromatin protein-γ regulates connective tissue growth factor by interacting with MMP-3, and MMP-3 knockdown suppresses connective tissue growth factor expression. These observations suggest that MMP-3 may be involved in the development, tissue remodelling, and pathology of arthritic diseases through regulation of connective tissue growth factor.[172]

MMP-3 may be involved in the development of arthritis, atherosclerosis, and tumour growth and metastasis.[173] Also, MMP-3 and VEGF levels decreased after tumor resection in patients with malignant tumors and increased in patients with recurrence, and therefore, could be of prognostic value in these patients.[174]

MMP-10

MMP-10 is expressed by macrophages and epithelium in response to injury, and its role in wound repair has been examined. In wounds of MMP-10 KO mice, collagen deposition and skin stiffness is increased, with no change in collagen expression or re- epithelialization. Increased collagen deposition in MMP-10 KO wounds was accompanied by less collagenolytic activity and reduced expression of specific metallocollagenases, particularly MMP-8 and -13, where MMP-13 was the key collagenase. Ablation and adoptive transfer approaches and cell-based models demonstrated that the MMP-10-dependent collagenolytic activity was a product of alternatively activated (M2) resident macrophages. These observations suggest a role for MMP-10 in controlling the tissue-remodeling activity of macrophages and moderating scar formation during wound repair.[175] MMP-10 may be involved in the transformation of normal oral epithelium to oral verrucous carcinoma and squamous cell carcinoma. MMP-10 expression levels are higher in oral squamous cell carcinoma than verrucous carcinoma, and therefore can be used in the differential diagnosis of the two tumors. [176] MMP-10 is limited to epithelial cells and may facilitate tumor cell invasion by targeting collagen, elastin, and laminin. Increased MMP-10 expression has been linked to poor clinical prognosis in some cancers decreased xenograft tumor growth, reduced angiogenesis, and apoptosis. These findings suggest that MMP-10 can play a role in tumor growth and progression, and MMP-10 inhibition may represent a rational strategy for cancer treatment.[177]

MMP-11

MMP-11 was first identified in stromal cells surrounding invasive breast carcinoma and has been proposed as one of the stroma-derived factors that play a role in the progression of epithelial malignancies.[178] Like all other members of the MMP gene family, stromelysin-3 is synthesized as an inactive precursor that must be processed to its mature form in order to express enzymatic activity. However, compared to other MMPs which require activation extracellularly, MMP-11 is secreted in its active form. MMP-11 can be processed directly to its enzymatically active form by an obligate intracellular proteolytic event that occurs within the constitutive secretory pathway.[179] In a study investigating the influence of genetic polymorphisms of MMP-
11 gene on the susceptibility to oral squamous cell carcinoma in a Taiwanese population, MMP-11 gene polymorphisms exhibited synergistic effects with the

environmental factors betel nut chewing and tobacco use on the susceptibility to oral squamous cell carcinoma. These observations suggest combined effects of MMP-11 gene polymorphisms and environmental carcinogens in the increased risk for oral squamous cell carcinoma and may be a predictive factor for tumor lymph node metastasis in Taiwanese with oral squamous cell carcinoma. The presence of MMP-11 in tumor tissues has suggested that it could promote cancer development by inhibiting apoptosis as well as enhancing migration and invasion of cancer cells. However, studies in animal models suggest that MMP-11 may play a negative role against cancer progression by suppressing metastasis.[180]

Matrilysins

MMP-7 plays a role in remodeling of tissues involved in development and reproduction such as the uterus, and could play a role in remodelling following tissue injury.[170]

MMP-26

As with MMP-7, MMP-26 lacks the hemopexin domain, believed to be involved in substrate recognition, and also the hinge region. MMP-26 mRNA is specifically expressed in the placenta and uterus. Recombinant MMP-26 demonstrates proteolytic activity toward several substrates including type IV collagen, β-casein, fibrinogen, fibronectin, gelatin, and vitronectin. MMP-26 also activates pro-MMP-9 (gelatinase B). The broad proteolytic activity and distribution of MMP-26 in different cell lines suggest that it may play a role in tissue-remodelling events associated with angiogenesis and tumor progression. MMP-26 expression may be linked to tumor invasion induced by GM-CSF. GM-CSF promotes tumor progression in different tumor models, and is associated with highly angiogenic and invasive tumors. [181-183]

Membrane-Type MMPs

MT-MMPs have membrane-anchoring domains and display protease activity at the cell surface, and therefore they are optimal pericellular proteolytic machines.[184] All MT-MMPs except MT4-MMP (MMP-17) can activate pro-MMP-2.13 MT1-MMP (MMP-14) activates pro-MMP-13 on the cell surface.[185]

MMP-14

MT1-MMP is ubiquitously expressed, binds TIMP-2, activates MMP-2, and stimulates cell migration in various cell types.[186] MMP-14 is best known for its collagenolytic activity, digesting type I (guinea pig), II (bovine), and III (human) collagens into characteristic 3/4 and 1/4 fragments. MT1- MMP may also degrade cartilage proteoglycan, fibronectin, laminin-1, vitronectin, α1-proteinase inhibitor, and α2-macroglobulin.[187] MT1-MMP induces activation of pro-MMP-2. In COS-1 cells, MT1-MMP could induce cell-surface binding of pro-MMP-2, which is consequently processed to an intermediate form Processing from the intermediate to the fully active form is dependent on MMP-2 concentration. Thus the MT1-MMP-induced cell-surface binding concentrates the MMP-2 intermediate form locally to allow autoproteolytic processing to the fully active MMP-2 form.[188] MT1-MMP could be an important molecular tool for cellular remodelling of the surrounding matrix. MT1-MMP has a major impact on invasive cell migration in both physiological and pathological settings such as immune cell extravasation or metastasis of cancer cells. Surface-associated MT1-MMP is able to cleave components of ECM, which is a prerequisite for proteolytic invasive migration.[189]

MMP-15

Like MT1-MMP, MT2- MMP localizes on the cell surface and mediates the activation of MMP- 2,which is associated with tumor invasion and metastasis. MT- MMPs are essential for pericellular matrix remodeling in late stages of development, as well as in growth and tissue homeostasis in postnatal life.[190]

MMP-16

MMP- 16 is a membrane-bound protein with a cytoplasmic tail. As a type I MT- MMP, MMP-16 could transform pro-MMP-2 to active MMP-2 and thereby facilitate tumor invasion. In patients with melanoma, increased expression of MMP-16 is associated with poor clinical outcome, collagen bundle assembly around tumor cell nests, and lymphatic invasion. MMP-16 enhances invasion of breast cancer cells.[191]

MMP-17

MMP-17 gene is expressed in a variety of human tissues mainly leukocytes, colon, ovary, testis, and the brain. The expression of MMP-17 in leukocytes together with its membrane localization suggest that it could be involved in activation of membrane-bound precursors of growth factors or inflammatory mediators such as TNF- α. MMP-17 transcripts are detected in all breast cancer cell lines, suggesting a role in tumor development/progression.[192]

MMP-24

MT- 24 is predominantly expressed in brain, kidney, pancreas, and lung. MMP- 24 can cleave pro-MMP-2 (progelatinase A) into its active MMP-2 form. MT5-MMP may contribute to the activation of pro-MMP-2 in tumor tissues, in which it is overexpressed, thereby facilitating tumor progression.[193] It is also highly expressed during embryonic development. In contrast to other MT-MMPs, MT5-MMP tends to shed from cell surface as soluble proteinases, thus offering flexibility as both a cell bound and soluble proteinase for ECM remodeling. Importantly, MT5-MMP regulates adult neural stem cell functional quiescence by cleaving and shedding of the N-cadherin ectodomain, supporting that the proliferative status of stem cells can be dynamically modulated by regulated cleavage of cell adhesion molecules.[194] MMP-24 is an essential modulator of neuroimmune interactions in thermal pain stimulation, and a mediator of peripheral thermal nociception and inflammatory hyperalgesia.[195] In a study investigating the expression of MMPs in different grades of human breast cancer tissues, mRNA expressions of MMP-1, -9, -11, -15, -24, and -25 were upregulated, while MMP-10 and -19 were downregulated in breast cancer compared with normal breast tissues. There was also a tumor grade-dependent increase in MMP-15 and -24 mRNA expression, supporting that MMPs are differentially regulated in breast cancer tissues and that they might play various roles in tumor invasion, metastasis, and angiogenesis.[196]

MMP- 25

MMP-25 is a GPI-anchored MMP that is highly expressed in leukocytes and some cancer tissues. MT6-MMP is present in lipid rafts and faces inward in living human polymorphonuclear leukocytes (PMNs), but translocates to the cell surface during neutrophil apoptosis.[197] PMNs express high levels of T6-MMP. MT6-MMP is present in the membrane, granules, and nuclear/endoplasmic reticulum/Golgi fractions of PMNs where it is displayed as a disulfide-linked homodimer of 120 kDa. Stimulation of PMNs results in secretion of active MT6-MMP into the supernatants. Membrane- bound MT6-MMP, conversely, is located in the lipid rafts of resting PMNs and stimulation does not alter this location. Interestingly, living PMNs do not display MT6- MMP on the cell surface. However, induction of apoptosis induces MT6-MMP relocation on PMNs' cell surface. Because of its localization in PMNs, MMP-25 may play a role in respiratory burst and IL-8 secretion.[199]

Conclusion

Considerable advancements have been made in the understanding of biochemical and structural aspects of MMPs, including their activation and catalytic mechanisms, substrate specificity, and the mechanism of inhibition by TIMPs.[200] In the classical view, MMPs are collectively capable of degrading all components of the extracellular matrix (ECM) and basement membrane, restricting their functions to tissue remodelling and maintenance.[201] However recent substrate identification studies reveal that MMPs are regulating the release or activation of chemokines, cytokines, growth factors, antibiotic peptides, and other bioactive molecules thus participating in physiological processes such as innate and adaptive immunity, inflammation, angiogenesis, bone remodelling, and neurite growth.[202] Apart from this , the increasing interest in MMP function also stems from their role in several pathological conditions, such as cancer or chronic inflammatory diseases.[203]

There is much evidence for the role of matrix metalloproteinases in the destructive processes of periodontal disease distinguishing them as a viable target for a chemotherapeutic approach. Since uncontrolled MMP activity can easily become destructive and lead to breakdown of homeostasis, it has been realised that their activity needs to be tightly regulated at different levels, through epigenetic, transcriptional and post-transcriptional control of gene expression, activation of their pro-enzymes, and inhibition of their activity.[201] The introduction of novel, adjunctive therapies to enhance the efficacy of existing mechanical procedures would contribute favourably to an integrated approach for the long-term, clinical management of periodontitis, particularly in susceptible patients, where a prolonged and excessive host response to the presence of bacteria promotes the activity of matrix metalloproteinases. Preclinical and clinical studies have demonstrated that inhibition of these matrix metalloproteinases, as a host modulatory approach, results in favourable changes in biochemical markers of the disease as well as clinical markers of therapeutic efficacy.[203] The application of targeted therapy toward MMP may serve as a useful adjunct to scaling and root planning .[204]

Matrix metalloproteinases have been found to play a major role in weakening the plaques formed with cardiovascular disease, leading to rupture and eventual thrombosis and infarction.[31] In diabetes, the same matrix metalloproteinases involved in the development of periodontitis as the sixth long-term complication of diabetes have also been associated with other well known complications of diabetes such as nephropathy, angiopathy, retinopathy and wound-healing problems.[205] Finally, periodontal disease has been found to put pregnant women at an increased risk of giving birth to preterm, low-weight babies. Matrix metalloproteinases have been found to play a role in the cervical effacement and dilation that precedes labor and are markers of risk for pre-term delivery since they are involved in pre-term premature rupture of the membranes playing a role in pre-term partuition.[206] In addition the dysregulation of MMP activities, especially in early cancer stages, raises great interest for MMPs as therapeutic targets in cancer treatment modalities. Clearly a matrix metalloproteinase inhibitor might not only help in the management of periodontitis, which has been associated with these systemic diseases, having an indirect effect on these processes but may also directly aid in the treatment and prevention of cardiovascular disease, diabetic complications and premature labors.[207]

MMPs are integrated in the network of multidirectional communication within tissues and cells as important regulators of cell proliferation and differentiation, tissue homeostasis, immune response and several other processes.[201] They are important components in many biological and pathological processes because of their ability to degrade ECM components. Therefore, it becomes important to understand their various roles in the body and the mechanisms behind tissue destruction to adopt a directed treatment approach.[202]

References

1. Reynolds JJ, Hembry RM, Meikle MC. Connective tissue degradation in health and periodontal disease and the roles of matrix metalloproteinases and their natural inhibitors. Adv Dent Res. 1994 Jul;8(2):312-9.

2. Quintero-Fabián S, Arreola R, Becerril-Villanueva E, Torres-Romero JC, Arana-Argáez V, Lara-Riegos J, Ramírez-Camacho MA and Alvarez-Sánchez ME (2019) Role of Matrix Metalloproteinases in Angiogenesis and Cancer. Front. Oncol. 9:1370.

3. Gross J, Lapiere CM. Collagenolytic activity in amphibian tissues: a tissue culture assay. Proc Natl Acad Sci USA 48: 1014–1022, 1962.

4. Reynolds JJ. Collagenases and tissue inhibitors of metalloproteinases: a functional balance in tissue degradation. Oral Dis. 1996 Mar;2(1):70-6.

5. Ryan ME, Ramamurthy S, Golub LM. Matrix metalloproteinases and their inhibition in periodontal treatment. Curr Opin Periodontol.

6. Reynolds JJ, Meikle MC. Mechanisms of connective tissue matrix destruction in periodontitis. Periodontol 2000. 1997 Jun;14:144-57.

7. Vu TH, Werb Z. Matrix metalloproteinases: effectors of development and normal physiology. Genes Dev. 2000 Sep 1;14(17):2123-33

8. Birkedal-Hansen H. Role of matrix metalloproteinases in human periodontal diseases. J Periodontol. 1993 May;64(5 Suppl):474-84

9. Ryan ME, Golub LM. Modulation of matrix metalloproteinase activities in periodontitis as a treatment strategy. Periodontol 2000. 2000 Oct;24:226-3810.

10. Malemud CJ. Matrix metalloproteinases (MMPs) in health and disease: an overview. Frontiers in Bioscience-Landmark. 2006 May 1;11(2):1696-701.

11. Hadler-Olsen E, Fadnes B, Sylte I, Uhlin-Hansen L, Winberg JO. Regulation of matrix metalloproteinase activity in health and disease. The FEBS journal. 2011 Jan;278(1):28-45.

12. Murphy G, Reynolds JJ. Extracellular matrix degradation. Connective Tissue and Its Heritable Disorders: Molecular, Genetic, and Medical Aspects. 2002 May 10:343-84.

13. Kinane DF. Regulators of tissue destruction and homeostasis as diagnostic aids in periodontology. Periodontology 2000. 2000 Oct;24(1):215-25.

14. Welgus HG, Stricklin GP. Human skin fibroblast collagenase inhibitor.

Comparative studies in human connective tissues, serum, and amniotic fluid. Journal of Biological Chemistry. 1983 Oct 25;258(20):12259-64.

15. Gross J, Lapiere CM. Collagenolytic activity in amphibian tissues: a tissue culture assay. Proceedings of the National Academy of Sciences. 1962 Jun;48(6):1014-22.

16. Nagai Y, Lapiere CM, Gross J. Tadpole collagenase. Preparation and purification. Biochemistry. 1966 Oct 1;5(10):3123-30.

17. Woessner JF. Catabolism of collagen and non-collagen protein in the rat uterus during post-partum involution. Biochemical Journal. 1962 May;83(2):304.

18. Woessner JF. MMPs and TIMPs—an historical perspective. Molecular biotechnology. 2002 Sep;22(1):33-49.

19. Collier IE, Wilhelm SM, Eisen AZ, Marmer BL, Grant GA, Seltzer JL, Kronberger AH, He CS, Bauer EA, Goldberg GI. H-ras oncogene-transformed human bronchial epithelial cells (TBE-1) secrete a single metalloprotease capable of degrading basement membrane collagen. Journal of Biological Chemistry. 1988 May 15;263(14):6579-87.

20. Okada Y, Morodomi T, Enghild JJ, Suzuki K, Yasui A, Nakanishi I, Salvesen G, Nagase H. Matrix metalloproteinase 2 from human rheumatoid synovial fibroblasts: purification and activation of the precursor and enzymic properties. European Journal of Biochemistry. 1990 Dec;194(3):721-30.

21. Galloway WA, Murphy GI, Sandy JD, Gavrilovic JE, Cawston TE, Reynolds

JJ. Purification and characterization of a rabbit bone metalloproteinase that degrades proteoglycan and other connective-tissue components. Biochemical Journal. 1983 Mar 1;209(3):741-52.

22. Okada Y, Nagase H, Harris Jr ED. Matrix metalloproteinases 1, 2, and 3 from rheumatoid synovial cells are sufficient to destroy joints. The Journal of rheumatology. 1987 May 1;14:41-2.

23. Lindsey ML, Zamilpa R. Temporal and spatial expression of matrix metalloproteinases and tissue inhibitors of metalloproteinases following myocardial infarction. Cardiovascular therapeutics. 2012 Feb;30(1):31-41.

24. Iyer RP, Patterson NL, Fields GB, Lindsey ML. The history of matrix metalloproteinases: milestones, myths, and misperceptions. American Journal of Physiology-Heart and Circulatory Physiology. 2012 Oct 15;303(8):H919-30.

25. Lovejoy B, Cleasby A, Hassell AM, Longley K, Luther MA, Weigl D, McGeehan G, McElroy AB, Drewry D, Lambert MH, Jordan SR. Structure of the catalytic domain of fibroblast collagenase complexed with an inhibitor. Science. 1994 Jan 21;263(5145):375-7.

26. Bode W, Reinemer P, Huber R, Kleine T, Schnierer S, Tschesche H. The X-ray crystal structure of the catalytic domain of human neutrophil collagenase inhibited by a substrate analogue reveals the essentials for catalysis and specificity. The EMBO journal. 1994 Mar;13(6):1263-9.

27. Stams T, Spurlino JC, Smith DL, Wahl RC, Ho TF, Qoronfleh MW, Banks TM, Rubin B. Structure of human neutrophil collagenase reveals large S1′ specificity pocket. Nature structural biology. 1994 Feb;1(2):119-23.

28. Maskos K. Crystal structures of MMPs in complex with physiological and pharmacological inhibitors. Biochimie. 2005 Mar 1;87(3-4):249-63.

29. Gooley PR, O'Connell JF, Marcy AI, Cuca GC, Axel MG, Caldwell CG, Hagmann WK, Becker JW. Comparison of the structure of human recombinant short form stromelysin by multidimensional heteronuclear NMR and X-ray crystallography. Journal of Biomolecular NMR. 1996 Jan;7(1):8-28.

30. Li J, Brick P, O'hare MC, Skarzynski T, Lloyd LF, Curry VA, Clark IM, Bigg HF, Hazleman BL, Cawston TE, Blow DM. Structure of full-length porcine synovial collagenase reveals a C-terminal domain containing a calcium-linked, four-bladed β-propeller. Structure. 1995 Jun 1;3(6):541-9

31. Jabłońska-Trypuć A, Matejczyk M, Rosochacki S. Matrix metalloproteinases (MMPs), the main extracellular matrix (ECM) enzymes in collagen

degradation, as a target for anticancer drugs. Journal of enzyme inhibition and medicinal chemistry. 2016 Nov 1;31(sup1):177-83.

32. Nagase H., Visse R., Murphy G. Structure and function of matrix metalloproteinases and TIMPs. Cardiovasc. Res. 2006;69:562–573.

33. Gialeli C, Theocharis AD, Karamanos NK. Roles of matrix metalloproteinases in cancer progression and their pharmacological targeting. The FEBS journal. 2011 Jan;278(1):16-27

34. Bilezikian JP, Raisz LG, Martin TJ, editors. Principles of bone biology.

Academic press; 2008 Sep 29.

35. Stetler-Stevenson WG, Krutzsch HC, Liotta LA. Tissue inhibitor of metalloproteinase (TIMP-2): a new member of the metalloproteinase inhibitor family. Journal of Biological Chemistry. 1989 Oct 15;264(29):17374-8.

36. Wilhelm SM, Collier IE, Marmer BL, Eisen AZ, Grant GA, Goldberg GI. SV40-transformed human lung fibroblasts secrete a 92-kDa type IV collagenase which is identical to that secreted by normal human macrophages. Journal of Biological Chemistry. 1989 Oct 15;264(29):17213-21.

37. Matrisian LM. The matrix-degrading metalloproteinases. Bioessays. 1992 Jul;14(7):455-63.

38. Matrisian, L.M., Glaichenhaus, N., Gesnel, M.C., Breathnach, R., 1985.

Epidermal growth factor and oncogenes induce transcription of the same cellular mRNA in rat fibroblasts. EMBO J. 4, 1435e1440.

39. .Matrisian LM, Glaichenhaus N, Gesnel MC, Breathnach R. Epidermal growth factor and oncogenes induce transcription of the same cellular mRNA in rat fibroblasts. The EMBO Journal. 1985 Jun;4(6):1435-40.

40. Hong SD, Hong SP, Lee JI, Lim CY. Expression of matrix metalloproteinase-2 and-9 in oral squamous cell carcinomas with regard to the metastatic potential. Oral oncology. 2000 Mar 1;36(2):207-13.

41. Okuda K, Miyazaki A, Momose M, Murata M, Nomura T, Kubota T, Wolff LF, Yoshie H. Lvels of tissue inhibitor of metalloproteinases-1 and matrix metalloproteinases-1 and-8 in gingival crevicular fluid following treatment with enamel matrix derivative (EMDOGAIN®). Journal of periodontal research. 2001 Oct;36(5):309-16.

42. Alpagot T, Bell C, Lundergan W, Chambers DW, Rudin R. Longitudinal evaluation of GCF MMP-3 and TIMP-1 levels as prognostic factors for progression of periodontitis. Journal of clinical periodontology. 2001 Apr;28(4):353-9.

43. Kiili M, Cox SW, Chen HW, Wahlgren J, Maisi P, Eley BM, Salo T, Sorsa T. Collagenase-2 (MMP-8) and collagenase-3 (MMP-13) in adult periodontitis: molecular forms and levels in gingival crevicular fluid and immunolocalisation in gingival tissue. Journal of clinical periodontology. 2002 Mar;29(3):224-32

44. Hrabec E, Strek M, Nowak D, Greger J, Suwalski M, Hrabec Z. Activity of type IV collagenases (MMP-2 and MMP-9) in primary pulmonary carcinomas: a quantitative analysis. Journal of cancer research and clinical oncology. 2002 Apr;128(4):197-204.

45. Kinane DF, Darby IB, Said S, Luoto H, Sorsa T, Tikanoja S, Mäntylä P. Changes in gingival crevicular fluid matrix metalloproteinase-8 levels during periodontal treatment and maintenance. Journal of periodontal research. 2003 Aug;38(4):400-4

46. Zhang L, Shi J, Feng J, Klocker H, Lee C, Zhang J. Type IV collagenase (matrix metalloproteinase-2 and-9) in prostate cancer. Prostate cancer and prostatic diseases. 2004 Dec;7(4):327-32.

47. Pesta M, Holubec L, Topolcan O, Cerna M, Rupert K, SEN LH, Treska V, Kormunda S, Elgrova L, Finek J, Cerny R. Quantitative estimation of matrix metalloproteinases 2 and 7 (MMP-2, MMP-7) and tissue inhibitors of matrix metalloproteinases 1 and 2 (TIMP-1, TIMP-2) in colorectal carcinoma tissue samples. Anticancer research. 2005 Sep 1;25(5):3387-91.

48. Emingil G, Tervahartiala T, Mãntylã P, Määttä M, Sorsa T, Atilla G. Gingival crevicular fluid matrix metalloproteinase (MMP)-7, extracellular MMP inducer, and tissue inhibitor of MMP-1 levels in periodontal disease. Journal of periodontology. 2006 Dec;77(12):2040-50.

49. Kumar MS, Vamsi G, Sripriya R, Sehgal PK. Expression of matrix metalloproteinases (MMP-8 and-9) in chronic periodontitis patients with and without diabetes mellitus. Journal of periodontology. 2006 Nov;77(11):1803-8.

50. Kopczyńska E, Dancewicz M, Kowalewski J, Makarewicz W, Kardymowicz H, Tyrakowski T. Usefulness of MMP-9/TIMP-1 ratio in estimation of lung cancer invasion and metastasis. Contemporary Oncology/Współczesna Onkologia. 2007;11(7):355-60.

51. Rysz J, Banach M, Stolarek RA, Pasnik J, Cialkowska-Rysz A, Koktysz R, Piechota M, Baj Z. Serum matrix metalloproteinases MMP-2 and MMP-9 and metalloproteinase tissue inhibitors TIMP-1 and TIMP-2 in diabetic nephropathy. Journal of nephrology. 2007 Jul 1;20(4):444-52.

52. Gürkan A, Emingil G, Saygan BH, Atilla G, Çınarcık S, Köse T, Berdeli A. Gene polymorphisms of matrix metalloproteinase-2,-9 and-12 in periodontal health and severe chronic periodontitis. archives of oral biology. 2008 Apr 1;53(4):337-45.

53. Bıyıkoğlu B, Buduneli N, Kardeşler L, Aksu K, Pitkala M, Sorsa T. Gingival Crevicular Fluid MMP-8 and– 13 and TIMP-1 Levels in Patients With Rheumatoid Arthritis and Inflammatory Periodontal Disease. Journal of Periodontology. 2009 Aug;80(8):1307-14.

54. Schumann C, Lepper PM, Frank H, 8Schneiderbauer R, Wibmer T, Kropf C, Stoiber KM, Rüdiger S, Kruska L, Krahn T, Kramer F. Circulating biomarkers of tissue remodelling in pulmonary hypertension. Biomarkers. 2010 Sep 1;15(6):523-32.

55. Rai B, Kaur J, Jain R, Anand SC. Levels of gingival crevicular metalloproteinases-8 and-9 in periodontitis. The Saudi dental journal. 2010 Jul 1;22(3):129-31.

56. Venkateshwari A, Sri Manjari K, Krishnaveni D, Nallari P, Vidyasagar A, Jyothy A. Role of plasma MMP 9 levels in the pathogenesis of chronic pancreatitis. Indian Journal of Clinical Biochemistry. 2011 Apr;26(2):136-9.

57. Reddy NR, Roopa D, Babu DM, Kumar PM, Raju CM, Kumar NS. Estimation of matrix metalloproteinase-3 levels in gingival crevicular fluid in periodontal disease, health and after scaling and root planing. Journal of Indian Society of Periodontology. 2012 Oct;16(4):549

58. 58. 13. Reddy NR, Deepa A, Babu DS, Chandra NS, Reddy CV, Kumar AK. Estimation of tissue inhibitor of matrix metalloproteinase-1 levels in gingival crevicular fluid in periodontal health, disease and after treatment. Journal of Indian Society of Periodontology. 2014 May;18(3):301.

59. Amato B, Coretti G, Compagna R, Amato M, Buffone G, Gigliotti D, Grande R, Serra R, de Franciscis S. Role of matrix metalloproteinases in non-healing venous ulcers. International Wound Journal. 2015 Dec;12(6):641-5.

60. Gupta N, Gupta ND, Gupta A, Khan S, Bansal N. Role of salivary matrix metalloproteinase-8 (MMP-8) in chronic periodontitis diagnosis. Frontiers of Medicine. 2015 Mar;9(1):72-6.

61. Ebersole JL, Nagarajan R, Akers D, Miller CS. Targeted salivary biomarkers for discrimination of periodontal health and disease (s). Frontiers in cellular and infection microbiology. 2015 Aug 19;5:62.

62. Arreguin-Cano JA, Ayerdi-Nájera B, Tacuba-Saavedra A, Navarro-Tito N, Dávalos-Martínez A, Emigdio-Vargas A, Barrera-Rodríguez E, Blanco-García N, Gutiérrez-Venegas G, Ventura-Molina E, León-Dorantes G. MMP-2 salivary activity in type 2 diabetes mellitus patients. Diabetology & Metabolic Syndrome. 2019 Dec;11(1):1-8.

63. Nardi GM, Cesarano F, Papa G, Chiavistelli L, Ardan R, Jedlinski M, Mazur M, Grassi R, Grassi FR. Evaluation of salivary Matrix Metalloproteinase (MMP-8) in periodontal patients undergoing non-surgical periodontal therapy and mouthwash based on ozonated olive oil: A randomized clinical trial. International journal of environmental research and public health. 2020 Sep;17(18):6619.

64. Sioustis IA, Martu MA, Aminov L, Pavel M, Cianga P, Kappenberg-Nitescu DC, Luchian I, Solomon SM, Martu S. Salivary metalloproteinase-8 and metalloproteinase-9 evaluation in patients undergoing fixed orthodontic treatment before and after periodontal therapy. International Journal of Environmental Research and Public Health. 2021 Feb;18(4):1583.

65. Liu J., Khalil R.A. Matrix Metalloproteinase Inhibitors as Investigational and Therapeutic Tools in Unrestrained Tissue Remodeling and Pathological Disorders. Prog. Mol. Biol. Transl. Sci. 2017;148:355–420

66. Maskos K. Crystal structures of MMPs in complex with physiological and pharmacological inhibitors. Biochimie. 2005;87:249–263.

67. Whittaker M., Floyd C.D., Brown P., Gearing A.J. Design and therapeutic application of matrix metalloproteinase inhibitors. Chem. Rev. 1999;99:2735– 2776

68. Rangasamy L., Geronimo B.D., Ortín I., Coderch C., Zapico J.M., Ramos A., de Pascual-Teresa B. Molecular Imaging Probes Based on Matrix Metalloproteinase Inhibitors (MMPIs) Molecules. 2019;24:E2982.

69. Cui N., Hu M., Khalil R.A. Biochemical and Biological Attributes of Matrix Metalloproteinases. Prog. Mol. Biol. Transl. Sci. 2017;147:1–73

70. Cerofolini L., Fragai M., Luchinat C. Mechanism and Inhibition of Matrix Metalloproteinases. Curr. Med. Chem. 2019;26:2609–2633

71. Verma R.P., Hansch C. Matrix metalloproteinases (MMPs): Chemical- biological functions and (Q)SARs. Bioorg. Med. Chem. 2007;15:2223–2268.

72. Klein T., Bischoff R. Physiology and pathophysiology of matrix metalloproteases. Amino Acids. 2011;41:271–290

73. Jacobsen J.A., Major Jourden J.L., Miller M.T., Cohen S.M. To bind zinc or not to bind zinc: An examination of innovative approaches to improved metalloproteinase inhibition. Biochim. Biophys. Acta. 2010;1803:72–94

74. Tsukada H., Pourmotabbed T. Unexpected crucial role of residue 272 in substrate specificity of fibroblast collagenase. J. Biol. Chem. 2002;277:27378– 27384.

75. Fischer T., Senn N., Riedl R. Design and Structural Evolution of Matrix Metalloproteinase Inhibitors. Chemistry. 2019;25:7960–7980

76. Murphy, G., Stanton, H., Cowell, S., Butler, G., Knäuper, V., Atkinson, S., & Gavrilovic, J. (1999). Mechanisms for pro matrix metalloproteinase activation. APMIS, 107(1-6), 38–44.

77. Van Wart HE, Birkedal-Hansen H. The cysteine switch: a principle of regulation of metalloproteinase activity with potential applicability to the entire

matrix metalloproteinase gene family. Proc Natl Acad Sci U S A. 1990; 87: 5578–5582.

78. Pei D, Weiss SJ. Furin-dependent intracellular activation of the human stromelysin-3 zymogen. Nature. 1995;375(6528):244–247.

79. English WR, Holtz B, Vogt G, Knauper V, Murphy G. Characterization of the role of the "MT-loop": an eight-amino acid insertion specific to progelatinase A (MMP2) activating membrane-type matrix metalloproteinases. J Biol Chem. 2001;276(45): 42018–42026.

80. Morgunova E, Tuuttila A, Bergmann U, Tryggvason K. Structural insight into them complex formation of latent matrix metalloproteinase 2 with tissue inhibitor of metalloproteinase 2. Proc Natl Acad Sci USA. 2002;99(11):7414– 7419.

81. Strongin AY, Collier I, Bannikov G, Marmer BL, Grant GA, Goldberg GI. Mechanism of cell surface activation of 72-kDa type IV collagenase. Isolation of the activated form of the membrane metalloprotease. J Biol Chem. 1995;270(10):5331–5338.

82. Sato H, Takino T, Kinoshita T, et al. Cell surface binding and activation of gelatinase A induced by expression of membrane-type-1-matrix metalloproteinase (MT1- MMP). FEBS Lett. 1996;385(3):238–240.

83. Kolkenbrock H, Orgel D, Hecker-Kia A, Noack W, Ulbrich N. The complex between a tissue inhibitor of metalloproteinases (TIMP-2) and 72-kDa progelatinase is a metalloproteinase inhibitor. Eur J Biochem. 1991;198(3):775–781.

84. Fridman R, Bird RE, Hoyhtya M, et al. Expression of human recombinant 72 kDa gelatinase and tissue inhibitor of metalloproteinase-2 (TIMP-2): characterization of complex and free enzyme. Biochem J. 1993;289(pt 2):411– 416.

85. Kucukguven A, Khalil RA. Matrix metalloproteinases as potential targets in the venous dilation associated with varicose veins. Curr Drug Targets. 2013;14(3):287–324.

86. Hollborn M, Stathopoulos C, Steffen A, Wiedemann P, Kohen L, Bringmann

A. Positive feedback regulation between MMP-9 and VEGF in human RPE cells. Invest Ophthalmol Vis Sci. 2007;48(9):4360–4367.

87. Mao D, Zhang Y, Lu H, Zhang H. Molecular basis underlying inhibition of metastasis of gastric cancer by anti-VEGFa treatment. Tumour Biol. 2014;35:8217–8223.

88. Cui Y, Sun YW, Lin HS, et al. Platelet-derived growth factor-BB induces matrix metalloproteinase-2 expression and rat vascular smooth muscle cell migration via ROCK and ERK/p38 MAPK pathways. Mol Cell Biochem. 2014;393(1–2): 255–263.

89. Rao VH, Kansal V, Stoupa S, Agrawal DK. MMP-1 and MMP-9 regulate epidermal growth factor-dependent collagen loss in human carotid plaque smooth muscle cells. Physiol Rep. 2014;2(2): e00224.

90. Page-McCaw A, Ewald AJ, Werb Z. Matrix metalloproteinases and the regulation of tissue remodelling. Nature reviews Molecular cell biology. 2007 Mar;8(3):221-33.

91. Vu TH, Shipley JM, Bergers G, Berger JE, Helms JA, Hanahan D, Shapiro SD, Senior RM, Werb Z. MMP-9/gelatinase B is a key regulator of growth plate angiogenesis and apoptosis of hypertrophic chondrocytes. Cell. 1998 May 1;93(3):411-22.

92. Colnot C, Sidhu SS, Balmain N, Poirier F. Uncoupling of chondrocyte death and vascular invasion in mouse galectin 3 null mutant bones. Developmental biology. 2001 Jan 1;229(1):203-14.

93. Colnot C, Thompson Z, Miclau T, Werb Z, Helms JA. Altered fracture repair in the absence of MMP9

94. Inada M, Wang Y, Byrne MH, Rahman MU, Miyaura C, López-Otín C, Krane SM. Critical roles for collagenase-3 (Mmp13) in development of growth plate cartilage and in endochondral ossification. Proceedings of the National Academy of Sciences. 2004 Dec 7;101(49):17192-7

95. Stickens D, Behonick DJ, Ortega N, Heyer B, Hartenstein B, Yu Y, Fosang AJ, Schorpp-Kistner M, Angel P, Werb Z. Altered endochondral bone development in matrix metalloproteinase 13-deficient mice.

96. Zhou Z, Apte SS, Soininen R, Cao R, Baaklini GY, Rauser RW, Wang J, Cao Y, Tryggvason K. Impaired endochondral ossification and angiogenesis in mice deficient in membrane-type matrix metalloproteinase I. Proceedings of the National Academy of Sciences. 2000 Apr 11;97(8):4052-7.

97. Chun TH, Sabeh F, Ota I, Murphy H, McDonagh KT, Holmbeck K, Birkedal- Hansen H, Allen ED, Weiss SJ. MT1-MMP–dependent neovessel formation

within the confines of the three-dimensional extracellular matrix. The Journal of cell biology. 2004 Nov 22;167(4):757-67.

98. Chantrain CF, Shimada H, Jodele S, Groshen S, Ye W, Shalinsky DR, Werb Z, Coussens LM, DeClerck YA. Stromal matrix metalloproteinase-9 regulates the vascular architecture in neuroblastoma by promoting pericyte recruitment. Cancer Research. 2004 Mar 1;64(5):1675-86.

99. Parks WC, Wilson CL, López-Boado YS. Matrix metalloproteinases as modulators of inflammation and innate immunity. Nature Reviews Immunology. 2004 Aug;4(8):617-29.

100. López-Boado YS, Wilson CL, Hooper LV, Gordon JI, Hultgren SJ, Parks WC. Bacterial exposure induces and activates matrilysin in mucosal epithelial cells. The Journal of cell biology. 2000 Mar 20;148(6):1305-15.

101. McGuire JK, Li Q, Parks WC. Matrilysin (matrix metalloproteinase-7) mediates E-cadherin ectodomain shedding in injured lung epithelium. The American journal of pathology. 2003 Jun 1;162(6):1831-43.

102. Haas TL, Madri JA. Extracellular matrix-driven matrix metalloproteinase production in endothelial cells: implications for angiogenesis. Trends in cardiovascular medicine. 1999 Apr 1;9(3-4):70-7.

103. Haro H, Crawford HC, Fingleton B, MacDougall JR, Shinomiya K, Spengler DM, Matrisian LM. Matrix metalloproteinase-3–dependent generation of a macrophage chemoattractant in a model of herniated disc resorption. The Journal of clinical investigation. 2000 Jan 15;105(2):133-41.

104. Wang M, Qin X, Mudgett JS, Ferguson TA, Senior RM, Welgus HG. Matrix metalloproteinase deficiencies affect contact hypersensitivity: stromelysin-1 deficiency prevents the response and gelatinase B deficiency prolongs the response. Proceedings of the National Academy of Sciences. 1999 Jun 8;96(12):6885-9.

105. D'Haese A, Wuyts A, Dillen C, Dubois B, Billiau A, Heremans H, Van Damme J, Arnold B, Opdenakker G. In vivo neutrophil recruitment by granulocyte chemotactic protein-2 is assisted by gelatinase B/MMP-9 in the mouse. Journal of Interferon & Cytokine Research. 2000 Jul 1;20(7):667-74.

106. Bhargava S , Lavanya R, Shalini B, Hiremath SK. Role of matrix-Metalloproteinases in the Pathogenesis of Periodontal Disease. EAS Journal of dentistry and oral medicine. 2020 March;2(2):46-51.

107. Rai B, Kharb S, Jain R, Anand SC. Biomarkers of periodontitis in oral fluids.Journal of oral science. 2008;50(1):53-6.

108. Özçaka Ö, Bıçakcı N, Pussinen P, Sorsa T, Köse T, Buduneli N. Smoking and matrix metalloproteinases, neutrophil elastase and myeloperoxidase in chronic periodontitis. Oral diseases. 2011 Jan;17(1):68-76.

109. Romanelli R, Mancini S, Laschinger C, Overall CM, Sodek J, McCulloch CA. Activation of neutrophil collagenase in periodontitis. Infection and immunity. 1999 May 1;67(5):2319-26.

110. Marcaccini AM, Meschiari CA, Zuardi LR, De Sousa TS, Taba Jr M, Teofilo JM, Jacob-Ferreira AL, Tanus-Santos JE, Novaes Jr AB, Gerlach RF. Gingival

crevicular fluid levels of MMP-8, MMP-9, TIMP-2, and MPO decrease after periodontal therapy. Journal of clinical periodontology. 2010 Feb;37(2):180-90.

111. Gursoy, U. K., Könönen, E., Pradhan-Palikhe, P., Tervahartiala, T., Pussinen,

P. J., Suominen- Taipale, L., & Sorsa, T. (2010). Salivary MMP-8, TIMP-1, and ICTP as markers of advanced periodontitis. Journal of clinical periodontology, 37(6), 487-493.

112. Makela M, Salo T, Uitto VJ, Larjava H. Matrix metalloproteinases (MMP-2 and MMP-9) of the oral cavity: cellular origin and relationship to periodontal status. Journal of dental research. 1994 Aug;73(8):1397-406.

113. HernándezRíos, M.; Sorsa, T.; Obregón, F.; Tervahartiala, T.; Valenzuela, M.A.; Pozo, P.; Dutzan, N.; Lesa_re, E.; Molas, M.; Gamonal, J. Proteolytic roles of matrix metalloproteinase (MMP)-13 during progression of chronic periodontitis: Initial evidence for MMP-13/MMP-9 activation cascade. J. Clin. Periodontol. 2009, 36, 1011–1017.

114. Beklen, A.; Tüter, G.; Sorsa, T.; Hanemaaijer, R.; Virtanen, I.; Tervahartiala, T.; Konttinen, Y.T. Gingival tissue and crevicular fluid co-operation in adult periodontitis. J. Dent. Res. 2006, 85, 59–63.

115. Marcaccini, A.M.; Novaes, A.B.; Meschiari, C.A.; Souza, S.L.; Palioto, D.B.; Sorgi, C.A.; Faccioli, L.H.; Tanus-Santos, J.E.; Gerlach, R.F. Circulating matrix metalloproteinase-8 (MMP-8) and MMP-9 are increased in chronic periodontal disease and decrease after non-surgical periodontal therapy. Clin. Chim. Acta 2009, 409, 117–122.

116. Mäntylä, P.; Stenman, M.; Kinane, D.; Salo, T.; Suomalainen, K.; Tikanoja, S.; Sorsa, T. Monitoring periodontal disease status in smokers and nonsmokers using a gingival crevicular fluid matrix metalloproteinase-8-specific chair-side test. J. Periodontal Res. 2006, 41, 503–512.

117. Mäntylä, P.; Stenman, M.; Kinane, D.F.; Salo, T.; Suomalainen, K.; Tikanoja, S.; Sorsa, T. Gingival cervicular fluid collagenase-2 (MMP-8) test stick for chair-side monitoring of periodontitis. J. Periodontal Res. 2003, 38,436–439.

118. Somerville, R.P.T.; Oblander, S.A.; Apte, S.S. Matrix metalloproteinases: Old dogs with new tricks. Genome Biol. 2003, 4, 216.

119. Loo, W.T.Y.; Wang, M.; Jin, L.J.; Cheung, M.N.B.; Li, G.R. Association of matrix metalloproteinase (MMP-1, MMP-3 and MMP-9) and cyclooxygenase- 2 gene polymorphisms and their proteins with chronic periodontitis. Arch. Oral Biol. 2011, 56, 1081–1090.

120. Santos, M.; Campos, M.; Souza, A.; Trevilatto, P.; Line, S. Analysis of MMP- 1 and MMP-9 promoter polymorphisms in early osseointegrated implant failure. Int. J. Oral Maxillofac. Implant. 2004, 19, 38–43.

121. Costa-Junior FR, Alvim-Pereira CC, Alvim-Pereira F, Trevilatto PC, De Souza AP, Santos MC. Influence of MMP-8 promoter polymorphism in early osseointegrated implant failure. Clinical oral investigations. 2013 Jan;17:311-6

122. Woolley DE, Roberts DR, Evanson JM (1975) Inhibition of human collagenase activity by a small molecular weight serum protein. Biochem Biophys Res Commun 66(2):747–754

123. Stetler-Stevenson WG, Brown PD, Onisto M cr 11 (1990). Tissue inhibitor of nietalloproteinases-2 (TIMP-2) mRNA expression in tumor cell lines and human tumor tissues. J Biol Chem 265: 13933-13938

124. Shapiro SD, Kobayashi DK, Welgus HG (1992b). Identification of TIMP-2 in human alveolar macrophages. Regulation of biosynthesis is opposite to that of metalloproteinases and TIMP-1. J Biol Chem 267: 13890-13894.

125. Pavloff N, Staskus PW, Kishnani NS ef al (1992). A new inhibitor of metalloproteinases from chicken: ChIMP-3. A third member of the TIMP family. J Bid Chem 267: 17321-17326

126. Leco KJ, Khokha R, Pavloff N et al (1994). Tissue inhibitor of metalloproteinases-3 (TIMP-3) is an extracellular matrix associated protein with a distinctive pattern of expression in mouse cells and tissues. J Biol Chern 269: 9352-9360.

127. Williamson RA, Marston FA, Angal S, Koklitis P, Panico M, Morris HR, Carne AF, Smith BJ, Harris TJ, Freedman RB. Disulphide bond assignment in human tissue inhibitor of metalloproteinases (TIMP). Biochem J. 1990;268:267–274.

128. Murphy G, Houbrechts A, Cockett MI, Williamson RA, O'Shea M, Docherty AJ. The N-terminal domain of tissue inhibitor of metallopro-teinases retains metalloproteinase inhibitory activity. Biochemistry. 1991;30:8097–8102.

129. Fernandez-Catalan C, Bode W, Huber R, Turk D, Calvete JJ, Lichte A, Tschesche H, Maskos K. Crystal structure of the complex formed by the membrane type 1-matrix metalloproteinase with the tissue inhibitor of

metalloproteinases-2, the soluble progelatinase A receptor. EMBO J. 1998;17:5238–5248.

130. Will H, Atkinson SJ, Butler GS, Smith B, Murphy G. The soluble catalytic domain of membrane type 1 matrix metalloproteinase cleaves the propeptide of progelatinase A and initiates autoproteolytic activation: regulation by TIMP-2 and TIMP-3. J Biol Chem. 1996;271: 17119–17123.

131. Page-McCaw A, Ewald AJ, Werb Z. Matrix metalloproteinases and the regulation of tissue remodelling. Nature reviews Molecular cell biology. 2007 Mar;8(3):221-33.

132. Eichler W, Friedrichs U, Thies A, Tratz C, Wiedemann P. Modulation of matrix metalloproteinase and TIMP-1 expression by cytokines in human RPE cells. Investigative ophthalmology & visual science. 2002 Aug 1;43(8):2767-73.

133. Meyer K, Ueberham E, Gebhardt R. Influence of organosulphur compounds from garlic on the secretion of matrix metalloproteinases and their inhibitor TIMP-1 by cultured HUVEC cells. Cell biology and toxicology. 2004 Jul;20:253-60.

134. Greenwald R. Tetracyclines may have potential benefit in rheumatoid arthritis but not for the reasons you think. J Clin Rheumatol 1995: 1: 185–189.

135. Galardy R, Grobelny D, Kortylewicz Z, Poncz L. Inhibition of human skin fibroblast collagenase by phosphorus-containing peptides. Matrix 1992: suppl 1: 259–262.

136. Schwartz M, Venkataraman S, Libby A, Mookhtiar K, Mallya S, Van Wart H, Birkedal-Hansen H. Sulfur-based inihibitors for matrix metalloproteinases. Matrix 1992: suppl 1: 309– 310.

137. Nagai Y, Hattori S, Odake S, Okayama T, Obata M, Morikawa T. Preparation of peptidyl hydroxamic acid derivatives which inhibit interstitial collagenases. Matrix 1992: suppl 1: 313.

138. Blundell T. Metalloproteinase super-families and drug design. Struct Biol 1994: 1: 73–75.

139. Fullmer H, Gibson W. Collagenolytic activity of gingivae of man. Nature 1966: 209: 728–729.

140. Golub, L.; Goodson, J.; Lee, H.; Vidal, A.; McNamara, T.; Ramamurthy, N.S. Tetracyclines Inhibit Tissue Collagenases: Effects of Ingested Low-Dose and Local Delivery Systems. J. Periodontol. 1985, 56, 93–97.

141. Golub, L.; Lee, H.; Ryan, M.; Giannobile, W.; Payne, P.; Sorsa, T. Tetracyclines inhibit connective tissue breakdown by multiple non-antimicrobial mechanisms. Adv. Dent. Res. 1998, 12, 12–26.

142. Uitto, V.; Firth, J.; Nip, L.; Golub, L. Doxycycline and chemically modified tetracyclines inhibit gelatinase A (MMP-2) gene expression in human skin keratinocytes. Ann. N. Y. Acad. Sci. 1994, 6, 140–151.

143. Sapna, G.; Gokul, S.; Bagri-Manjrekar, K. Matrix metalloproteinases and periodontal diseases. Oral Dis. 2014, 20, 538–550.

144. Steinsvoll, S. Periodontal disease, matrix metalloproteinases and chemically modified tetracyclines. Microb. Ecol. Health Dis. 2004, 16, 1–7.

145. Chung L, Dinakarpandian D, Yoshida N, et al. Collagenase unwinds triple- helical collagen prior to peptide bond hydrolysis. EMBO J. 2004;23(15):3020– 3030.

146. Mittal R, Patel AP, Debs LH, et al. Intricate functions of matrix metalloproteinases in physiological and pathological conditions. J Cell Physiol. 2016;231(12):2599–2621.

147. Ayuk SM, Abrahamse H, Houreld NN. The role of matrix metalloproteinases in diabetic wound healing in relation to photobiomodulation. J Diabetes Res. 2016;2016:2897656.

148. Chen X, Thibeault SL. Role of tumor necrosis factor-alpha in wound repair in human vocal fold fibroblasts. Laryngoscope. 2010;120(9):1819–1825.

149. Shimizu Y, Kondo S, Shirai A, Furukawa M, Yoshizaki T. A single nucleotide polymorphism in the matrix metalloproteinase-1 and interleukin-8 gene promoter predicts poor prognosis in tongue cancer. Auris Nasus Larynx. 2008;35(3):381–389.

150. Mizrachi A, Koren R, Hadar T, Yaniv E, Morgenstern S, Shvero J. Expression of MMP-1 in invasive well-differentiated thyroid carcinoma. Eur Arch Otorhinolaryngol. 2011;268(1):131–135.

151. Hasty KA, Pourmotabbed TF, Goldberg GI, et al. Human neutrophil collagenase. A distinct gene product with homology to other matrix metalloproteinases. J Biol Chem. 1990;265(20):11421–11424.

152. Knauper V, Murphy G, Tschesche H. Activation of human neutrophil pro- collagenase by stromelysin 2. Eur J Biochem. 1996;235(1–2):187–191.

153. Nwomeh BC, Liang HX, Diegelmann RF, Cohen IK, Yager DR. Dynamics of the matrix metalloproteinases MMP-1 and MMP-8 in acute open human dermal wounds. Wound Repair Regen. 1998;6(2):127–134.

154. Gutierrez-Fernandez A, Inada M, Balbin M, et al. Increased inflammation delays wound healing in mice deficient in collagenase-2 (MMP-8). FASEB J. 2007;21(10):2580–2591.

155. Lee W, Aitken S, Sodek J, McCulloch CA. Evidence of a direct relationship between neutrophil collagenase activity and periodontal tissue destruction in vivo: role of active enzyme in human periodontitis. J Periodontal Res. 1995;30(1):23–33.

156. Dalvie D, Cosker T, Boyden T, Zhou S, Schroeder C, Potchoiba MJ. Metabolism distribution and excretion of a matrix metalloproteinase-13 inhibitor, 4-[4-(4 fluorophenoxy)-benzenesulfonylamino]tetrahydropyran-4- carboxylic acid hydroxyamide (CP-544439), in rats and dogs: assessment of the metabolic profile of CP-544439 in plasma and urine of humans. Drug Metab Dispos. 2008;36(9): 1869–1883.

157. Wang G, Zhang Y, Zhao X, Meng C, Ma L, Kong Y. MicroRNA-411 inhibited matrix metalloproteinase 13 expression in human chondrocytes. Am J Transl Res. 2015;7(10):2000–2006.

158. Mashimo Y, Sakurai-Yageta M, Watanabe M, et al. Induction of the matrix metalloproteinase 13 gene in bronchial epithelial cells by interferon and identification of its novel functional polymorphism. Inflammation. 2016;39(3):949–962.

159. Chen JH, Tsai CH, Lin HY, et al. Interleukin-18 is a pivot regulatory factor on matrix metalloproteinase-13 expression and brain astrocytic migration. Mol Neurobiol. 2016;53(9):6218–6227.

160. You Y, Shan Y, Chen J, et al. Matrix metalloproteinase 13-containing exosomes promote nasopharyngeal carcinoma metastasis. Cancer Sci. 2015;106(12):1669–1677. Steffensen B, Wallon UM, Overall CM. Extracellular matrix binding properties of recombinant fibronectin type II-like modules of human 72-kDa gelatinase/type IV collagenase. High affinity binding to native type I collagen but not native type IV collagen. J Biol Chem. 1995;270(19):11555–11566.

161. Shipley JM, Doyle GA, Fliszar CJ, et al. The structural basis for the elastolytic activity of the 92-kDa and 72-kDa gelatinases. Role of the fibronectin type II- like repeats. J Biol Chem. 1996;271(8):4335–4341.

162. Koyama H, Iwata H, Kuwabara Y, Iwase H, Kobayashi S, Fujii Y. Gelatinolytic activity of matrix metalloproteinase-2 and -9 in oesophageal carcinoma; a study using in situ zymography. Eur J Cancer. 2000;36(16):2164–2170.

163. Aimes RT, Quigley JP. Matrix metalloproteinase-2 is an interstitial collagenase.

Inhibitor-free enzyme catalyzes the cleavage of collagen fibrils and soluble native type I collagen generating the specific 3/4- and 1/4-length fragments. J Biol Chem. 1995;270(11):5872–5876..

164. Murray GI, Duncan ME, O'Neil P, McKay JA, Melvin WT, Fothergill JE. Matrix metalloproteinase-1 is associated with poor prognosis in oesophageal cancer. J Pathol. 1998;185(3):256–261.

165. Talvensaari-Mattila A, Paakko P, Turpeenniemi-HujanenT. Matrixmetalloproteinase-2 (MMP-2) is associated with survival in breast carcinoma. Br J Cancer. 2003;89(7): 1270–1275.

166. Nam SI, Kwon TK. Dexamethasone inhibits interleukin-1beta-induced matri metalloproteinase-9 expression in cochlear cells. Clin Exp Otorhinolaryngol. 2014;7(3): 175–180.

167. Tomlinson ML, Garcia-Morales C, Abu-Elmagd M, Wheeler GN. Three matrix metalloproteinases are required in vivo for macrophage migration during embryonic development. Mech Dev. 2008;125(11–12):1059–1070.

168. Koyama H, Iwata H, Kuwabara Y, Iwase H, Kobayashi S, Fujii Y. Gelatinolytic activity of matrix metalloproteinase-2 and -9 in oesophageal carcinoma; a study using in situ zymography. Eur J Cancer. 2000;36(16):2164–2170.

169. Pei D, Weiss SJ. Furin-dependent intracellular activation of the human stromelysin-3 zymogen. Nature. 1995;375(6528):244–247.

170. Verma RP, Hansch C. Matrix metalloproteinases (MMPs): chemical-biological functions and (Q)SARs. Bioorg Med Chem. 2007;15(6):2223–2268.

171. Hollborn M, Stathopoulos C, Steffen A, Wiedemann P, Kohen L, Bringmann

A. Positive feedback regulation between MMP-9 and VEGF in human RPE cells. Invest Ophthalmol Vis Sci. 2007;48(9):4360–4367.

172. Eguchi T, Kubota S, Kawata K, et al. Novel transcription-factor-like function of human matrix metalloproteinase 3 regulating the CTGF/CCN2 gene. Mol Cell Biol. 2008;28(7):2391–2413.

173. Ye S, Watts GF, Mandalia S, Humphries SE, Henney AM. Preliminary report: genetic variation in the human stromelysin promoter is associated with progression of coronary atherosclerosis. Br Heart J. 1995;73(3):209–215.

174. Kolomecki K, Stepien H, Bartos M, Kuzdak K. Usefulness of VEGF, MMP-2, MMP-3 and TIMP-2 serum level evaluation in patients with adrenal tumours. Endocr Regul. 2001;35(1):9–16

175. Rohani MG, McMahan RS, Razumova MV, et al. MMP-10 regulates collagenolytic activity of alternatively activated resident macrophages. J Invest Dermatol. 2015;135(10):2377–2384.

176. Kadeh H, Saravani S, Heydari F, Keikha M, Rigi V. Expression of matrix metalloproteinase-10 at invasive front of squamous cell carcinoma and verrucous carcinoma in the oral cavity. Asian Pac J Cancer Prev. 2015;16(15):6609–6613.

177. Zhang G, Miyake M, Lawton A, Goodison S, Rosser CJ. Matrix metalloproteinase-10 promotes tumor progression through regulation of angiogenic and apoptotic pathways in cervical tumors. BMC Cancer. 2014;14:310.

178. Basset P, Bellocq JP, Wolf C, et al. A novel metalloproteinase gene specifically expressed in stromal cells of breast carcinomas. Nature. 1990;348(6303):699– 704.

179. Pei D, Weiss SJ. Furin-dependent intracellular activation of the human stromelysin-3 zymogen. Nature. 1995;375(6528):244–247.

180. Zhang X, Huang S, Guo J, et al. Insights into the distinct roles of MMP-11 in tumor biology and future therapeutics (Review). Int J Oncol. 2016;48(5):1783– 1793.

181. Uria JA, Lopez-Otin C. Matrilysin-2, a new matrix metalloproteinase expressed in human tumors and showing the minimal domain organization required for secretion, latency, and activity. Cancer Res. 2000;60(17):4745–4751.

182. de Coignac AB, Elson G, Delneste Y, et al. Cloning of MMP-26. A novel matrilysin like proteinase. Eur J Biochem. 2000;267(11):3323–3329.

183. Marchenko GN, Ratnikov BI, Rozanov DV, Godzik A, Deryugina EI, Strongin AY. Characterization of matrix metalloproteinase-26, a novel metalloproteinase widely expressed in cancer cells of epithelial origin. Biochem J. 2001;356(pt 3):705–718.

184. Sohail A, Sun Q, Zhao H, Bernardo MM, Cho JA, Fridman R. MT4-(MMP17) and MT6-MMP (MMP25), a unique set of membrane-anchored matrix metalloproteinases: properties and expression in cancer. Cancer Metastasis Rev. 2008; 27(2):289–302.

185. Knauper V, Will H, Lopez-Otin C, et al. Cellular mechanisms for human procollagenase-3 (MMP-13) activation. Evidence that MT1-MMP (MMP-14) and gelatinase a (MMP-2) are able to generate active enzyme. J Biol Chem. 1996;271(29): 17124–17131.

186. Radichev IA, Remacle AG, Shiryaev SA, et al. Biochemical characterization of the cellular glycosylphosphatidylinositol-linked membrane type-6 matrix metalloproteinase. J Biol Chem. 2010;285(21):16076–16086.

187. Ohuchi E, Imai K, Fujii Y, Sato H, Seiki M, Okada Y. Membrane type 1 matrix metalloproteinase digests interstitial collagens and other extracellular matrix macromolecules. J Biol Chem. 1997;272(4):2446–2451.

188. Butler GS, Butler MJ, Atkinson SJ, et al. The TIMP2 membrane type 1 metalloproteinase "receptor" regulates the concentration and efficient activation of progelatinase A. A kinetic study. J Biol Chem. 1998;273(2):871–880.

189. Wiesner C, El Azzouzi K, Linder S. A specific subset of RabGTPases controls cell surface exposure of MT1-MMP, extracellular matrix degradation and three- dimensional invasion of macrophages. J Cell Sci. 2013;126(pt 13):2820–2833.

190. Sato H, Seiki M. Membrane-type matrix metalloproteinases (MT-MMPs) in tumor metastasis. J Biochem. 1996;119(2):209–215.

191. Liu J, van Mil A, Aguor EN, et al. MiR-155 inhibits cell migration of human cardiomyocyte progenitor cells (hCMPCs) via targeting of MMP-16. J Cell Mol Med. 2012;16(10):2379–2386.

192. Puente XS, Pendas AM, Llano E, Velasco G, Lopez-Otin C. Molecular cloning of a novel membrane-type matrix metalloproteinase from a human breast carcinoma. Cancer Res. 1996;56(5):944–949.

193. Llano E, Pendas AM, Freije JP, et al. Identification and characterization of human MT5-MMP, a new membrane-bound activator of progelatinase a overexpressed in brain tumors. Cancer Res. 1999;59(11):2570–2576.

194. Porlan E, Marti-Prado B, Morante-Redolat JM, et al. MT5-MMP regulates adult neural stem cell functional quiescence through the cleavage of N-cadherin. Nat Cell Biol. 2014;16(7):629–638.

195. Folgueras AR, Valdes-Sanchez T, Llano E, et al. Metalloproteinase MT5-MMP is an essential modulator of neuro-immune interactions in thermal pain stimulation. Proc Natl Acad Sci USA. 2009;106(38):16451–16456.

196. Benson CS, Babu SD, Radhakrishna S, Selvamurugan N, Ravi SB. Expression of matrix metalloproteinases in human breast cancer tissues. Dis Markers. 2013;34(6): 395–405.

197. Fortin CF, Sohail A, Sun Q, McDonald PP, Fridman R, Fulop T. MT6-MMP is present in lipid rafts and faces inward in living human PMNs but translocates to the cell surface during neutrophil apoptosis. Int Immunol. 2010;22(8):637–649.

198. Zhao H, Sohail A, Sun Q, et al. Identification and role of the homodimerization interface of the glycosylphosphatidylinositol-anchored membrane type 6 matrix metalloproteinase (MMP25). J Biol Chem. 2008;283(50):35023–35032.

199. Fortin CF, Sohail A, Sun Q, McDonald PP, Fridman R, Fulop T. MT6-MMP is present in lipid rafts and faces inward in living human PMNs but translocates to the cell surface during neutrophil apoptosis. Int Immunol. 2010;22(8):637–649.

200. Robert Visse and Hideaki Nagase Function, and Biochemistry Matrix Metalloproteinases and Tissue Inhibitors of Metalloproteinases: Structure,

201. Lo¨ffek S, Schilling O, Franzke C.W. Biological role of matrix metalloproteinases: a critical balance. European Respiratory Journel. 2011 Jul 1;38(1): 191-208

202. Lopez-Otin C, Matrisian LM. Emerging roles of proteases in tumour suppression. Nat Rev Cancer 2007; 7: 800–808.

203. Page-McCaw A, Ewald AJ, Werb Z. Matrix metalloproteinases and the regulation of tissue remodelling. Nat Rev Mol Cell Biol 2007; 8 221–233.

204. Sapna G, Gokul S, Bagri-Manjrekar K. Matrix metalloproteinases and periodontal diseases. Oral diseases. 2014 Sep;20(6):538-50.

205. Taiyeb-Ali TB, Raman RP, Vaithilingam RD. Relationship between periodontal disease and diabetes mellitus: an Asian perspective. Periodontology 2000. 2011 Jun;56(1):258-68

206. Bobetsis YA, Graziani F, Gürsoy M, Madianos PN. Periodontal disease and adverse pregnancy outcomes. Periodontology 2000. 2020 Jun;83(1):154-74.

207. Giannobile WV. Host-response therapeutics for periodontal diseases. Journal of periodontology. 2008 Aug;79:1592-600.

FSC
www.fsc.org
MIX
Papier | Fördert
gute Waldnutzung
FSC® C083411

Kolibri 360 GmbH
Ferdinand-Jühlke-Straße 7
99095 Erfurt, Deutschland
produktsicherheit@kolibri360.de

Druck:
CPI Druckdienstleistungen GmbH
im Auftrag der
Kolibri 360 GmbH
Ferdinand-Jühlke-Str. 7
99095 Erfurt